Keto Mastery

Follow the Advanced Ketogenic/ Low Carbohydrate Diet That Many Top Performing Men and Women Athletes Have Used for Reaching Peak Performance By Following This Complete Dieting Guide!

By Georgia Bolton

Table of Contents

3. Ketosis is free reign to stuff your craw with deep-fried butter and pork belly

4. Nutrient proportions are set in stone

5. Ketosis is a risk factor for ketoacidosis

6. Ketosis is the ultimate, final way to lose weight

7. Ketosis is a high protein diet

8. Ketosis destroys your heart and valves

9. Keto can cause flu-like symptoms

10. Ketosis exacerbates fatty liver

11. Ketosis carries out a systematic extermination of your gut flora

12. Any fat is good fat

And so it is written

Chapter 11: Good Foods

Fats and oils

Meat, poultry, and seafood

Nuts, Seeds, Legumes, etc.:

Fruits:

Vegetables:

Dairy

Snacks:

Drinks:

Foods to avoid, or at least eat in moderation:

Fats:

Meats:

Starches

Fruits

Vegetables

Sugars, sweeteners, desserts, etc.

Snacks

Drinks:

Conclusion

Introduction

The public consciousness is bubbling with all manner of diets and weight loss strategies - from intermittent fasting to the Atkins diet to the Paleo diet. The one that seems to be continuously mysterious to a lot of people is the ketogenic diet, or keto, for short. Is it a high protein, high fat diet? Low carb diet? Neither of these - the keto diet is based on the principle of changing the body from a carbohydrate-powered metabolic engine to a fat-powered one. The name "ketogenic" comes from the compounds that are the end result of the breakdown of fatty acids in the liver when there is not enough sugar in the bloodstream, called ketones. When blood glucose is low, either via fasting or by a particular diet, the body breaks down stored fat into ketones as fuel.

Now how does all this apply to the diet? Essentially, the ketogenic diet is one that revolves around the high-fat intake, moderate protein intake, and very low-carbohydrate intake to keep your body in a state of "ketosis" - burning ketones for fuel instead of sugar.

Interestingly, the genesis of the ketogenic diet lies in the treatment of epilepsy. Treatises from ancient Greece going back as far as 400 BCE prescribe the use of fasting to treat seizures. Obviously, they didn't know it, but fasting bodies created ketones to fuel themselves. In the early 20th century, Rollin Turner Woodyatt used it to treat epileptic patients with some success. In the 1990s, it received national attention again as a treatment for epilepsy, and from there, the diet gained momentum and other similar diets emerged such as the Atkins diet and Paleo diet.

How do the keto, Atkins, and the paleo diet differ from each other, you may ask? If you look into a nutrition magazine, you'll be up to your eyeballs with those three and a thousand more strategies.

To keep it concise, keto and Atkins are fairly similar. The primary difference is that the goal of Keto is to put you in ketosis, a metabolic state of burning ketones for fuel, while Atkins is centered around strictly weight loss. Atkins also is more structured in its approach, classically containing four different "stages" and which are based around time and amount of weight lost. Finally, and most notably, the Atkins diet is more generous in its carbohydrate consumption.

The paleo diet revolves around trying to recreate a hypothetical "caveman" diet of unprocessed foods, composed primarily of organic protein and vegetables. What's more important to the paleo diet is the particular food choices, not necessarily a delicate balance of fat, protein, and carbohydrates.

The paleo diet has a lot in common with other diets, in that it emphasizes whole food choices over processed ones, and usually ethically-sourced ones at that, but does not really concern itself with macronutrient balance and ketosis.

Ketosis is a big subject, with many facets to consider, from how it fixes the modern diet to what to eat. If you're interested in changing your energy systems, read on. The knowledge in this book should put you on the path to a more informed and healthier version of yourself.

Chapter 1: The Problems with the Modern Diet

As many people are probably already aware, we are in the midst of something that can be described aptly as a global metabolic crisis. Obesity, heart disease, and type-2 diabetes rates are higher than ever before and still climbing, not only in the developed world but even in burgeoning countries. The reason for this is simply too massive a topic to be covered in this book, but what it comes down is nutritional havoc perpetrated by excessive simple carbohydrate consumption. When you eat simple carbs, they are easily broken down by body into their component sugars, which causes the pancreas to release insulin, which stores some of those component sugars as glycogen in the muscle and liver, to be used as immediate, quick-to-access energy, and the rest to be deposited in our fat cells, making us to balloon up. In addition, they amongst the easiest to acquire and rewarding foods known to man, being cheap, widely available, and versatile. Simple carbohydrates cover a range from the more commonly known choices like candy and doughnuts, typically what someone thinks of when they hear "simple" or "bad" carbs, to daily staples like bread, rice, and pasta.

Theoretically, if one entered a prolonged state of carb withdrawal, a fast or diet composed primarily of fat and protein, your body does what it naturally does - consumes the stored carbohydrates in your body, the glycogen in your muscles and liver, for energy and then starts tapping into the fat cells for sustenance - ketosis. The problem is, our modern world, we never get to this point. Our world is one where food is widely available, and the quickest, cheapest, easiest, and most rewarding things to eat are carbohydrates, forestalling your ketogenic state forever unless one makes the conscious and informed choice to enter it.

One of the problems is in the United States especially, for most of the 20th century, there was a strong backlash against dietary fat based on faulty science that started long, destructive love affair with carbohydrates that we're still collectively getting over. The term "fat" to refer to lipids was probably one of the worst things PR wise that could have happened to them, as the association was obvious - fat makes you fat. That's the most natural conclusion in the world to make, right? Well, human metabolism is never that simple, and the maxim of "fat is the enemy" has been simply destructive on our collective health. Carbohydrates are also inherently less filling than fats, meaning one has to consume more of them to attain the same satiety that fat does. It's true that fat has a higher calorie per gram count, nine per gram, about double carbohydrate's four per gram, so satiety one feels is much greater, usually leading one to consume fewer calories at the end of the day. That's another advantage of the keto diet; you'll be feeling so satisfied from your diet that there's no longer a need to accidentally consume 400 calories in chips or other snacks.

With that in mind, ever looked at the calorie count on a can of soda or a glass of fruit juice? They're almost always in excess of 100, all packed it into a neat little can or bottle and does nothing for actual feelings of hunger, and these products are EVERYWHERE. In the case of fruit juice, it's being marketed as healthy even though almost all the things that keep fruit from being a metabolic insulin bomb have been stripped away.

Despite the huge prevalence of these sorts of foods everywhere, the idea of "fat is the enemy" still has a decent amount of weight behind it (no pun intended); think about how many products you see marketing themselves as healthier and better for you for being low in fat - in reality, if you want to send your body's fat-burning systems into overdrive, consuming fat and avoiding carbs is the headspace you want to be in.

Unfortunately, today we live in a fast-paced world where convenience is king and the quicker something can be done, the better. This has led to an increase in processed foods, foods artificially preserved with harmful chemicals and stripped of all base nutritional content in the process. In fact, with a lot of foods, including white flour, white rice, and pasta, nutrients have to be added back in to make sure that people don't suffer from certain deficiencies that would be easy to avoid in a world of whole foods. The other unfortunate reality is that almost every single processed food is packed to the brim with sugar, and in the case of things like pastries, are also made of insulin spiking white flour.

Processed foods high in oil always take the cheapest possible way out, with oil that's cheap to produce and heavily processed in of itself, usually a saturated fat or, even worse, trans fats. Trans fats are hydrogenated vegetable fats and are easy to store for a long time and melt at temperatures considered desirable, and are commonly used in things like mass-produced pastries and fast food.

What does hydrogenated mean? To properly get ahold of this, one needs to understand the chemical structure of fats. Fats have long chains of bonded hydrogen and carbon when bonded together once, they're called saturated, and twice, they're called unsaturated. Hydrogenation is simply the process of changing an unsaturated (liquid at room temperature, canola, peanut, or corn oil) fat to a saturated (Solid at room temperature, think butter, lard, or coconut oil) one by changing the chemical bonds of carbon from double to single. What are the ramifications of all these chemical shenanigans for your body? They end up increasing the amount of "bad" cholesterol, LDLs and drop the amount of "good" cholesterol, HDLs, increase triglycerides in blood, and increase inflammation all around the body. These sorts of oils are found nearly everywhere, in almost every processed and fast food, and, as mentioned before, convenience is king. People are on the run, people are busy, and are more interested in temporarily squashing hunger pangs than the long-term implications of their diet and food choices. Instead of fixing a simple and filling meal at home that is high in protein and healthy fats, people are opting for the simpler choice.

How to Fix It

What can be done to remedy the modern diet? The good thing about today's world is that healthy food is cheaper than ever, and the internet acts as a veritable infinite library of information for every food under the sun, and the ones still buried. It just takes a trained eye and a mind well trained in proper decisions about "whole" foods. For the sake of this book, take whole foods to mean unprocessed meats, wild seafood, raw dairy, fresh fruit and vegetables, dried beans, and minimally processed, whole grains.

Following the keto diet isn't a prerequisite for health, but mindfulness about your food choices is, and that's where everyone should start. To start assessing how badly the modern diet has blown out your body, a mental note should be made of what you eat and be diligent to change what needs to be changed. It's not a simple process - renovating any part of your life is never easy - but the simplest place to start is possibly in identifying any food choices that stick out to you as bad. We all know the ones that claw at the back of our minds – the guilty pleasures, the "convenience" foods, the elaborate coffees that are basically desserts that we're all so fond of, things you know it would be best for you to cut out. That's where this book starts, just trying to get you to be more cognizant of what you eat, to take the first step and eliminate some of the choices that you know are bad for you, the foods that are helping you to pack on an extra layer of fluff for winter, despite the fact that there's a good chance you won't be spending it in a cave. Once that first step is taken, the rest can follow suit so much easier.

Setting goals is always a good idea, be it financially, professionally, personally, or fitness wise. Goals give you a sense of illuminating purpose, and, in a way, light a path for you to follow along to your destination. Start small and get bigger – is your goal to eat more fiber, protein, to put on healthy weight, or to lose bad weight? Once you have a goal in mind, more serious planning can occur. You base your food choices around what you want to mold your body into.

Getting Informed

To properly fix the train wreck that is the modern diet, one needs to know how exactly to implement healthier choices. This is a neglected aspect of modern education for many people, despite how absolutely essential to health and happiness it is. We live in an age where there is more information freely circulating about any topic you can imagine, yet for some reason, this information has failed to properly diffuse across the modern consciousness. It's no wonder that in an age where processed, artificially crafted foods are so common and cheap, people, in their woeful ignorance, are forsaking actual healthy choices, which is causing diabetes, obesity and heart disease to run rampant.

To get a basic gestalt of the different nutrients, a short guide will be provided here:

- Carbohydrates: Energy, the most bioavailable fuel source. Made up of sugars; bread, pasta, rice, beans, starchy vegetables, and other grains
- Fat/Lipids: Stored energy of plants and animals, made of a glycerin molecule with fatty acids attached. High satiety. Vegetable oils, butter, lard.
- Proteins: Structural component of living tissue, helps maintain and build tissues. Composed of amino acids. Meat, fish, eggs, dairy products, and tofu.
- Fiber: Indigestible carbohydrate necessary for gut health, keeps hunger and blood sugar in check. Found in unprocessed whole grains (Whole wheat pasta, bread, brown rice) beans, fruits, and vegetables
- Vitamins and Minerals: Two distinct micronutrients, meaning they're needed in small amounts, for various body functions such as muscle action, digestion, eye health, and dozens of other roles.

This brings us nicely into the next point; fiber is *extremely* important for satiety and keeping blood sugar stable. Sudden spikes in blood sugar cause it to be stored as fat by insulin and the feared "sugar crash," getting sleepy after polishing off a plate of pasta or bowl of rice.

Simple Versus Complex Carbohydrates

This is probably a term you've heard before, but doubtless, the true meaning is somewhere floating in a metaphorical miasma around your (and millions of other's) minds. Simple carbs are easily broken down by the body and spike the blood sugar. That fact was touched on earlier in this chapter, but it neglected to define a complex carb. Complex carbs are not as refined as simple ones, they don't have their fiber, and nutritious bits stripped away, and because of that, they are harder for your body to break down, don't spike your blood sugar and cause you to feel full longer. If one desires to be healthier, complex is the way to go.

They keep cravings off and keep your belly feeling full and happy for hours after, as well as maintaining their micronutrient profile of vitamins and minerals. The USDA recommended fiber intake for adults is between 20 and 30, and that's easy to get when your diet is filled with things like vegetables, fruit, whole grain bread, pasta, brown rice, and beans. Common knowledge also dictates that vegetables are absolutely essential for health for other reasons, they are full of antioxidants and are among the most micronutrient dense foods on earth, not counting chunks of animals some would consider rather unpalatable, namely liver, kidneys, sweetbreads, and the like.

Fats and Proteins

While fiber is important for satiety, your body can't run off it. Fat helps keep you fueled, and if you get it from healthy animal sources, grass-fed beef and butter, heritage pigs, and monounsaturated oils like olive oil, coconut oil, and avocado, there's nothing to be feared in terms of hidden health dangers. Protein is also essential for maintaining your living tissue, keeping your hundreds of muscles and organs maintained and strong.

In times of ketosis, whether via fasting or conscious decision, protein is broken via gluconeogenesis (Gluco = sugar, Neo = New, Genesis = Creation) to fuel the brain, as well as being used to maintain body composition, and keeping you full. This makes protein something you can't afford to neglect, keto diet or not.

Fats come in a few different flavors – monounsaturated, polyunsaturated, trans, and saturated. Monounsaturated are your "good fats," liquid at room temperature fats like olive, almond, and avocado oil, and are composed of numerous heart-healthy fatty acids and usually have other micronutrients as well. Polyunsaturated are not as good for you, but not necessarily bad, corn, canola, soybean oil. They can still be good for the body, but not as much as their monounsaturated brothers. Trans fats are to be avoided at all costs due to a serious link with heart disease. The most mysterious sibling of the fat family is saturated fat, solid at room temperature. Animal fats and coconut oil – depending on the quality of the source (Happier animals or virgin coconut oil) saturated fat can have serious health benefits, from hormone regulation to omega-3s, but it might impact your blood lipid levels, depending on genes, diet, and activity levels. Don't cut it out altogether, but try not to make dinner lard with a side of coconut oil.

Putting it all Together

Now that the information has been passed to you, it's relatively easy to start putting a diet together to remedy the many problems of the modern diet. While a ketogenic diet is going to be the main focus of the rest of this book, it can be hard for a lot of people to go full keto, and the point of this chapter was more to elucidate you on basic diet choices. A healthy panacea to the modern dietary disaster would be a diet with little to no simple carbohydrates, only coming from fruit if possible, high in complex carbs in the form of vegetables and whole grains and beans. The rest should be built from healthy, sustainable proteins and fats to keep you full, happy, and functional. Buying expensive organic products isn't necessary, and oftentimes they aren't necessarily better for you, just containing a slightly different micronutrient profile. What's more important for your immediate health is keeping a good macronutrient profile rich in fiber, vitamins, and minerals.

Chapter 2: The Good Parts of Keto

Keto has been espoused across by people in all walks of life as a powerful tool to lose weight, improve athletic performance, reduce brain fog, control cravings and increase self-control, lower insulin resistance, control certain diseases, and even save money and time.

Keto and Weight Loss

To learn how the ketogenic diet helps you lose weight, one must first visualize how the body stores its excess energy – as fat. All the fat on the human body, or adipose tissue, represents a huge reservoir of potential energy, that could last us up to weeks. What happens with a lot of people is that that fat never really gets tapped in to, as the continuous flow of carbs into the body defeats the need for the body to break into its supply. When you starve your body of carbohydrates, it turns to its stored fat for fuel, a state of ketosis, producing ketones. Ketones are like the backup generator for your body, produced in the liver, and triggered by low blood sugar. Lipase, an enzyme, cleaves off some of the stored triglycerides, and they're chauffeured off on a silver platter for your liver to break down and use as energy.

Ketones manifest in three types, all of which are somewhat hard to pronounce and spell: acetoacetate, acetone, and beta-hydroxybutyrate. The first one is important as it can be used to test your levels of ketosis, and the last two are what enters your body cells and becomes energy, beta-hydroxybutyrate being the best ketone for energy. All these molecules are taken from body fat, which can only be accessed once muscle glycogen reaches a certain depletion point. What happens is your body is essentially eating itself in the way it was designed to do, by burning through its fat reserves; it's theorized that in the past, our ancestors, hunter-gatherers, lived in a way very similar to this, as access to fresh game didn't necessarily happen every day.

The nature of how ketosis shreds the fat off your body is also interesting. For some reason yet unknown to metabolic scientists, ketosis has shown to be able to reduce the abdominal fat – fat around our viscera, our organs, better than traditional weight loss programs. This means the organs can work easier and be more free of inflammation, sparing them some of the stress that leads to type-2 diabetes, heart problems, and veritable cornucopia of other maladies. Our overall lipid profile changes as well, with a stark decline in triglycerides, reduction in LDLs, and increase in HDLs being among the most commonly observed phenomena.

One of the more "quiet" or unsung benefits of going on a ketogenic diet is the fact that the longer you stay on it, the more efficient your body gets at producing ketones and supplying you with energy from the thousands of calories stashed in your fat cells. This is the reason why many people are trying it out for the first-time crash and give up; it's not necessarily an easy or expedient thing for your body to go from a glucose-fueled system to a fat-fueled system. It takes your metabolism a while to catch up to what your mind is putting it through, but after it gets adapted, your body is rendered into a biological fat combustion engine. In addition, because your diet is composed of "heavier" foods, fats and proteins, you can feel full in what is ultimately less food and fewer calories, eliminating a need to snack and controlling your cravings. Numerous studies have proven the effectiveness of the diet, in 2012 a study conducted on obese kids and teenagers found reduced body weight, fat mass, and waist size and a reduction in shrinkage insulin levels, meaning that what they eat containing carbs won't immediately be shuttled off into their fat cells. Another study in 2017 found that a group while combining the diet with a CrossFit exercise regime, lost an average of 6 pounds of fat and improved their athletic ability over a period of six weeks.

Improved Mental Focus

Everyone and their mother's dog has gone through the stage of sleepy, heavy-headedness that accompanies consuming a whole large pizza with a side of cheesy bread and a marinara sauce with as much sugar as candy - the feared high blood sugar crash that can make it feel like you're wading through concrete. Augmented ability to cut through brain fog and focus on the task at hand is a commonly reported symptom for people in ketosis, likely explained by the fact that they're no longer in a constant, brutal cycle of eating and crashing and eating and crashing. Beta-hydroxybutyrate, one of the most important ketone bodies, might be partially responsible for this, as when it barges into your brain in all its energy-rich glory, it stimulates the growth of new mitochondria. Obviously, it can't be conclusively linked to abated feelings of fogginess, but it may explain how the diet has helped people with epilepsy, covered below.

Keto and Chronic Diseases

The original formulation for the ketogenic diet was as a way to combat epilepsy, but also has shown some success in treating maladies like diabetes, heart disease, Alzheimer's and some cancers.

The keto diet and epilepsy have shared a bed for quite some time, as that was the reason it was first brought into being. The exact mechanism of action is still poorly understood, but research at John Hopkins University shows that for children, who, for one reason or another, can't be placed on anticonvulsants, can have their seizure incidents reduced by 50% in half of the test subjects and by 90% in a third of patients. The best explanation put forth as of yet as to how it effectively sabotages epilepsy is that ketones themselves are anticonvulsant, via the fact that they are more energy efficient than glucose. The neurons in the brain adapt and increase the number of mitochondria, the powerhouse of the cell that produces energy. The increased number of mitochondria can more easily handle the massive increased energy load that flows through the brain during a seizure.

Type-2 diabetes also lays within the sights of keto's metabolic sniper rifle by draining the sugar from your blood and reducing your need for insulin and diabetes-controlling medication. To fully grasp the breadth of this, insulin resistance needs to better understood. When your cells become insulin resistant, they start refusing to take in the glucose-insulin is trying to shove into its doors, so it stays in the blood. When this happens, the pancreas goes bonkers and makes more insulin, making you a person with diabetes. A lowered insulin resistance means your body can take in the sugar like it's supposed to and your body goes back to normal.

In a study performed in 2008, over the course of 24 weeks, diabetic patients on a ketogenic diet nearly exterminated their need for medication, with 95.2% of them versus a mere 62% who were put on a low-glycemic diet. Their HDL ("Good" cholesterol) also increased, while the low-glycemic group experienced no change, and lost about 10 more pounds, losing on average 25 while the low-glycemic lost 15.

Heart disease is also treated by keto, simply because it is often linked to carrying excess weight around, which a state of ketosis helps to eliminate. In addition, inflammation from excessive carbohydrate intake, the bane of any well-functioning circulatory system, drops, freeing up huge amounts of stress on the heart and its various tendrils and valves. It should be important to note that for best heart-disease countering effects of keto; one should make sure that a higher portion of the fat they're consuming come from monounsaturated than saturated as it is rich in omega-3s, which is a great boon for the heart.

Alzheimer's Disease is a progressive form of slow dementia, usually seen in the elderly. While assuredly not a panacea for the disease that ruins lives of not only those suffering from it but from their families, certain attributes of keto can help alleviate symptoms. It has been found in animals with it that it can improve proprioception – balance, and coordination, and when supplementing with ketone esters, can reduce amyloid plaque, a characteristic marker of the disease. Again, the exact mechanism of action isn't known, and research is still ongoing. Areas of pathologic neurology are still poorly understood, probably because neurology itself is poorly understood.

Finally, some cancers, particularly brain cancers seem to respond to ketogenic diets. The theory is that the lowered blood sugar and insulin levels may reduce global inflammation, as inflammation has been known to be a root cause in many diseases. A slew of case studies found it aiding treatment of glioblastoma multiforme. Unfortunately both the most widespread and aggressive form of noggin cancer one can acquire. It is interesting to note that the diet shares a certain number of traits with fasting, most obviously autophagy, or "self-eating," the burning of fat for fuel, and both have shown some success in shrinking tumors. Perhaps it is the combination of what is basically starving out the cancer cells of easy to access energy along with the reduced global inflammation.

Oxidative stress, the accumulation of highly reactive molecules in the body without enough compounds to properly neutralize them, has been shown to lead to an increase in global inflammation. Inflammation has been linked time and time again with a slew of chronic diseases, the classical killers – diabetes, heart disease, and cancer. Antioxidants work to detoxify these free radicals; common sources are fruit and vegetables. One very interesting find was that when consuming carbohydrates alone, the body essentially switches off its natural system for handling oxidative stress, necessitating the consumption of antioxidant-rich foods. But when forsaking carbohydrates and consuming dietary fat and protein, these natural antioxidant systems are still switched on. The implications of this are immense, as it could radically change the way we look at our diets and the consumption of carbohydrates from here on out. With this in mind, it's no surprise that a diet that reduces systemic inflammation is also one that has shown some success in shutting down diseases whose root lays in inflammation.

Ketosis and Athletic Performance

Ketosis can be great for athletes of a certain type as well as people simply trying to lose weight. In particular, the ketogenic diet may be the perfect fit for endurance athletes - long-distance runners, cyclists, rowers, and swimmers. To understand why an understanding of basic exercise energy systems is important. For athletes involved in more "start and stop" type activities -- football players, wrestlers, rugby players, where one goes from 0% effort to 110% maximal effort that lasts more than 10 seconds, more easily accessible sources of energy are needed in the form of carbohydrates stored as glycogen in the muscle. Glycogen can be accessed by the body much more readily, as it's a form of energy designed for sudden powerful movements, so it's of much more use by athletes in explosive, short bouts with recovery time. High-intensity interval training, in other words. Endurance exercise is a more "steady state" form of exercise, a slow burn, so to speak. It's not particularly intense, but ideally, there are little to no breaks. The more stable nature of endurance sports lets the body chip off fat as it needs it for a slower burn activity. What may happen to a lot of runners who fuel themselves up on carbohydrates is a crash – they start out strong, running hard and fast, and then once their initial stores deplete, they're hitting a wall and lagging behind. The steady delivery of ketones to muscles keeps this problem from occurring.

Take this with a grain of salt, as a state of ketosis, when first adjusting to it, might leave some feeling sapped of energy. It's important to give yourself time to adjust before going off and trying to run the same marathon that Pheidippides ran 2500 years ago. In addition, even after achieving a state of steady ketosis where usual activities don't destroy you, to give yourself "trial runs" of a lighter exercise load than you're used to give your muscles and connective tissue time to adapt under exercise stress.

Ketosis, Food Choices, and Saving Money

One of the "soft" benefits of ketosis is thus – it lets you enjoy a rich, "regal" diet, the stuff that people usually consider the "heart" of the meal because of its wholeness and filling nature - foods like butter, meat, fish, other animal products, nuts, and whole fat dairy. Most of your calories will come from here by necessity, as they are the most fat-rich sources of nutrients unless you're interested in chugging olive oil. As a quick aside, taking shots of olive oil is not a wholly unheard-of tactic as a more extreme method of getting more healthy monounsaturated fat and filling your caloric need for the day.

When was the last time you found someone chowing down on a huge bowl of plain rice or pasta and considered it a decadent treat? And while this is a "soft" benefit, enjoying your calories from these rich and real foods without the sense of guilt that might sometimes accompany them, there is also a more "solid" benefit. It's been proven time and time again that appetites are suppressed on a low carb diet, a diet higher in protein and fat will end with you eating fewer calories. In addition, once you get used to eating a keto diet, it will be more than enough to keep your cravings for snacks away. If your diet consists of almost strictly fats, and you end up eating less of it, you'd save money on a grocery bill. In addition, you'd no longer have a desire to snack, between your body becoming more used to taking advantage of its fat stores and the fact that eating 800 calories of meat, fish, or eggs sits heavier than 800 calories of bread. In a way, this will save you time and money as well, and we all know time is money and money is time, as there's no stopping at a convenience store to pick up an expensive-per-the-calorie snack.

Wrapping It All Up

Keto's power as a diet is impressive, helping people lose weight, reduce chronic inflammation and thus fight many diseases that are ravaging our bodies, help us run, swim, row, and bike longer, and letting us enjoy a rich diet without the guilt while saving us time and money.

Chapter 3: The Bad Parts of Keto

Unfortunately, there is nothing that does not cast a shadow, metaphorical or otherwise, and ketosis has its fair share of downsides that must be considered before taking the plunge into a whole new metabolic world.

A Delicate Balance

A ketogenic diet is typically calorically broken down as 75% fat, 20% protein, and 5% carbohydrates, this is the approximate proportion – it changes depending on the person and their needs. Knowing this is all fine and dandy, but implementing it is a harder quest that requires a level of dietary dedication not seen in many people most of the time. It calls for a level of micromanagement many people are simply not willing to invest their time into, and because of this, it can be a major reason the diet fails.

Counting calories is one thing, measuring precise percentages of carbs, fats, and proteins is another. This delicate balance, if upset, will throw off the entire metabolic reaction, and, if done more incorrectly, can lead to more serious medical implications. A single miscount can throw the body out of ketosis and lead one to feel distressed and discouraged. This sort of thinking is not only hard to get into, but also hard to maintain, most medical professionals recommend that a keto diet only be maintained for a one to three months at max to take advantage of its fat-burning potential, before switching to a more "regular" diet.

Unfortunately, this can lead to Yo-yo effect, when one quickly regains the weight they lost when switching to a new diet. This is potentially more disastrous than simply being overweight, as the trauma the yo-yo effect puts on the body has been linked to increased mortality. It's not a secret that many doctors recommend that before starting a keto diet that they're consulted to test the initial health, so something needlessly tragic and avoidable doesn't happen. Oftentimes doctors recommend routine testing of ketone bodies during the diet and especially if one intends to follow it for an extended period, but that is something that can easily be done at home with the proper equipment. It's also always a good idea to talk with a nutritionist to find out the optimal macronutrient balance for you, how many calories you need in a day so you can find out how much of each nutrient you should be getting per day, and the right kinds of foods to eat while on it. Someone with a history of heart disease may want to avoid excessive saturated animal fat consumption, for instance. The overarching reality is that the ketogenic diet requires a lot of management and balancing, which many people may not be prepared to deal with.

Dietary Restrictions and Expenses

This is probably where most people falter and break, where its strength becomes its weakness. While keto does let you essentially eat, guilt-free, some of the richest foods known to man, variety is the spice of life, and if food and cooking is a major part of your life and sacrificing it isn't an option, keto simply may not be the right choice for you. It may be both a blessing and a curse that modern society has offered us such a wealth of different food that we can try at virtually any time – if we were a bunch of starving hunter-gatherers, keto would be the reality instead of merely one road that might be followed. A world without pasta, rice, bread, and candy might be too much for certain people, especially athletes who are used to fueling themselves up on such foods.

Should you be able to get over your relative scarcity of ingredients, there's the issue of "I don't know if I can whip up interesting ways to eat meat/coconut/eggs/oils/veggies 7 days a week, 3 times a day. That's a LOT of meals to come up with not a lot of ingredients, especially if you aren't interested in the culinary arts. For these people, there simply may not be enough interesting ways to eat keto and keep it up.

Cost is also to be considered. Optimally, a keto diet is one filled with healthy animal fats, foods like avocados, fresh vegetables, and olive and coconut oil. The problem with this is that for those of us who aren't dedicated to the art of savings, this can get expensive quick. It was said in the previous chapter that keto CAN save you money, the caveat here is that it CAN save you money, it potentially can, once you get used to it – if you get used to it, and still, some people simply have larger appetites than others and can eat 36 oz of steak a day and be ready for dessert afterward. If meat was once a thing you did a few times a week, having a bit of chicken breast here or there and maybe a steak or pork chops every now and then, this author finds that it can quickly burn a hole in your pocket. If you don't know how to look for deals and learn to love what's on sale, then this may be impossible for you. And if you don't have the knack to shop right and still crave variety, one might be tempted to branch into a few new hobbies, hunting, and fishing, to get your daily fat and protein needs.

The mere fact that the keto diet limits variety massively may impede many people from ever reaching ketosis in the first place, much less being able to maintain it for any significant length of time. Unfortunately, this is fundamental to the diet, as the minute you eat enough carbs to stop ketosis, you are no longer following the keto diet. While these problems with ketosis cannot be avoided, with proper supervision, there is a variety that can be, which will be covered next.

The "Keto Flu"

The transition from a carb-burning machine to a fat burning machine, especially when your body has been essentially never had the chance to do the latter before, can be a little traumatic for your biology. The keto flu is a collection of – you guessed it – flu-like symptoms that is a unique sort of misery our bodies make us suffer through as punishment for such a drastic change from what it's used to. Not everyone goes through it, but those that do feel like it's 1918 and the Spanish Flu is all the pathological rage again. It's analogous to what a heroin or nicotine addict goes through, but for carbohydrates, minus all the terrifying hallucinations and feelings of impending death (In the heroin addict's case more so than the nicotine addict's case), in other words - withdrawal.

Suffering can be mild to severe and vary by the day, making this truly "keep you on the edge of your seat" sort of misery, and can last from days to weeks. Symptoms can range to any of the following unpleasantries: nausea, vomiting, diarrhea, rapacious cravings for sugar, unexplained muscle soreness and cramping, insomnia, reduced ability to focus, stomach and abdominal cramps, dizziness, feelings of weakness, irritability, and headaches. In other words, a veritable garden of earthly delights. Thankfully, nothing lasts forever, and the keto flu is relatively harmless if one knows how to treat it.

As tempting as it may be to run a marathon or enter an impromptu cage fighting match while vomiting last night's dinner of steak with a side of coconut milk and steamed broccoli into the nearest bowl-shaped receptacle, avoiding strenuous exercise is crucial so your body can adapt to its new fuel source. Along with this is staying hydrated, as that can really help abate the feelings of cramps and help replace any fluids that may have been forced out one of your many orifices.

Along with the water, what is also lost during violent purging at one or both ends are electrolytes. Sodium, potassium, calcium, and magnesium are absolutely critical to keeping yourself on this planet as a functional human being, keeping you at a level strong enough that your boss doesn't decide to fire you for your manufactured "keto flu" disease. A loss of electrolytes can also seriously impact the kidneys in some of the most unpleasant ways imaginable, the damage can can lead to the dreaded kidney stone. Also, and less dramatically but more worrisome, overall kidney damage. Magnesium is especially essential as it assists in soothing muscle pain and ushering you off into the dreamworld. With that in mind, as in all things, getting enough sleep is also vital. Sleep is where your body makes little adjustments and modifications and repairs to assure that it is running at peak capacity, where it fixes all the damage you've done to it during the day. Without adequate sleep, doubtless one will ever fully be able to transition to a ketogenic lifestyle or even any kind of productive and healthy one.

Ketogenic Diets Can Impair Athletic Ability and Promote Muscle Wasting

For any meatheads reading this, this can be a terrifying prospect. The unfortunate reality is, as mentioned earlier, is that not every sport is designed for ketosis. Not all sports are slow burn cardio; in fact, not even most are! Many are more explosive, requiring high amounts of speed and power as well as maximal effort. Here is where ketosis lags behind – as you're barely eating any carbs, your body can't store the intramuscular glycogen it uses for fast, powerful athletic movements. What this equates to is being weaker in the field, in the weight room, or on the mats, and feeling fatigued quicker. Even if you do somehow manage to induce a shamanic trance where pain and exhaustion are mere tricks of devilish spirits, there is still the fact that adequate amounts of muscle glycogen are needed for recovery, meaning that this diet in its traditional build is not optimal for athletes. There are, of course, modifications, but this current discussion only takes into account a "traditional" ketogenic diet.

The next and more serious negative implication of ketosis is the fact that your brain cannot survive off of ketone bodies alone. The brain requires around 400 calories a day to function, around 100 grams of glucose, more if you're a genius and less if you're missing some marbles (this statement not scientifically supported). Your liver is very good at manufacturing that glucose that you need from your diet, when keto is done right, providing just enough protein and carbohydrates to be broken down into glucose to fuel your brain. The scary part happens when you miscount either of those two nutrients, undereat both of them, and eat TOO much fat, as your brain can give an executive order to your liver to start wasting away muscle tissue, which is then converted into glucose to keep itself alive. This is a relatively easy thing to avoid, as only around four ounces of protein a day are needed to avoid this, but the prospect is there.

The Possibility of Ketoacidosis

Ketoacidosis is when the count of ketones in your bloodstream reaches pathological and dangerous levels, usually only seen in a certain form of diabetes. What happens is the excessive amount of ketones turns your blood acidic, which gets deadly fast as your body exists within a very narrow pH range. The reality is that unless you really poorly mismanage your keto diet, you probably won't end up here, but it is a potential side effect that can affect your liver, brain, and kidneys. If you're following the keto diet, and someone thinks your breath smells like a strawberry that joined a street gang (In less colorful language, a "bad" sort of fruity) this can be a sign of ketoacidosis, as you exhale acetones produced by your liver. Other symptoms are pleasantries like thirst, urination, abdominal pain and vomiting, and disorientation. If you go through this, get yourself to the ER immediately because the reaper will come otherwise.

Is It Right For You?

With all of the potential failings of the keto diet now laid bare for the world and the reader to see, a necessary question must be asked: Is the ketogenic diet right for me? It can be a powerful weight management tool if used well, capable of providing scores of other health benefits that would lead to a long and happy life. But also, it's a sensitive beast, and if implemented poorly it can lead to a slew of negative symptoms. It's not for everyone, the serious athlete, the enthusiastic chef, those of us who lack the attention span and eye for detail necessary for keeping ketosis maintained and not falling off, are not necessarily good candidates, unless modifications in both the diet and lifestyle are consciously made.

Chapter 4: Getting Started with Ketosis

Now that there are no more mysteries as to what a keto diet is, its good and its bad parts, and have decided that it's right for you, you can move on to actually implement a ketogenic diet in your day-to-day life.

There's a Chinese proverb that is often abused by various motivational speakers and unengaging middle school teachers; "the journey of a thousand miles begins with a single step." Despite how tired and seemingly used up this proverb is, there is wisdom in it, as the hardest part of beginning anything new is to start doing it in the first place. Once you start something, it almost seems easier to continue. Your mental landscape shifts from "I don't even want to start it" to "I've started it, I may as well finish it," and building this kind of basic resolve is important with making a hard lifestyle change like keto, especially when it's as pervasive as it is.

Ask Yourself Why

In the first chapter, I talked about how when you're trying to get yourself off the poison of modern western diets; it's important to have a goal in mind, as it effectively serves as a road through the tangled darkness. When making a goal, one of the best ways to go about it is to approach it systematically, ask yourself questions until you know EXACTLY what you'll be doing and when, whittle your goal down like you're a man wrongly imprisoned, and the only way to pass the time is to carve chess pieces from pieces of soft rock.

In the case of this goal setting system, set yourself an overarching goal. For instance, the usual reasons for going on ketosis are "I want to lose weight," but others could include "I want to improve my endurance performance," or "I want to manage my diabetes." These are obviously vague, open goals, but that's good because there's room to grow, room to focus. This brings us to the next question in the system; "Where am I right now?" How much do you weigh right now? What is your time for a 5k right now? How many shots of insulin keeps you breathing? Once you have a reference point, you can then riddle yourself with the questions "What do I want my 5k time to be?" "How much fat do I want to lose?" "How much do I want to rely on my diabetes medication moving ahead?" Ask yourself these questions to get a more concrete handle on your goal. Once you have that figured out, you've pulled back to where you are, right now, in this current moment, you can start assessing how far you are from your goal and setting realistic steps, and take it day to day.

What changes can you make every day to reach your goal and make it a reality?

Tracking your goals

As much as we can plan and scheme, life comes at us one day at a time, so making sure that you're making these active changes in your life every day is how you're going to get where you want to go. Recording is always a good idea; if it wasn't, our scientific procedures would still be done via guesstimations and "close enough!" Recording lets you look at things from above and track your goals day to day, and from there week to week, letting you set manageable markers of progress for yourself, and then get a good idea of how long it will take you to get there. Recording must become a habit, a thing you've essentially beat into your subconscious via force of will. As an aside, there's interesting find in behavioral neurology that boils down to "Humans are most happy when they can see they are making progress on a goal, not upon reaching the goal itself."

Example plan for weight loss:

My goal is to lose weight.

How much do you weight right now?

180 pounds.

How much weight do you want to lose?

20 pounds.

How will you get there?

By following a ketogenic diet, which will put my body in a state of fat-burning ketosis, fill me heavy foods that drive down my total calorie intake and prevent me from snacking.

Okay, that sounds good. After one week of following this diet, how much have you lost? You logged it in, I hope!

2 pounds.

If you're doing this right and nothing drastic happens (losing a leg, etc.) you should be there in 10 weeks, give or take.

Another, for cardiovascular endurance:

My goal is to improve my 5k time.

What is your current 5k time?

30 minutes.

How much do you want to improve it?

By 8 minutes

How will you get there?

A ketogenic diet will help me because of the slow and steady nature of my sport, the slow burn release of energy from fat-burning ketosis fits very well as an energy system, by forsaking more carbohydrates, I avoid the carbohydrate-induced energy crash and can keep a steadier, but overall faster time.

Okay, sounds solid. After one week, how has your time improved? You've been writing it down, right?

By 1 minute.

So, reasonable, unless nothing drastic happens (again, loss of a leg may impede the ability to run somewhat) you should get there in 8 weeks, give or take.

Note: Neither of these plans is designed to be comprehensive weight loss or athletic plans, they are merely depicted here to get an idea of an efficient way to structure your goals so you can reach them.

Actually Getting Started With Ketosis

Now that that song and dance is done with, your goals are properly illuminated, and you've gotten an idea how much you'll progress per week and how keto will help you, you can move on to the meat of the problem, that being getting started with eating a ketogenic diet and living the "lifestyle."

Breaking it down:

The most important step with starting a ketogenic diet is knowing how much of each macronutrient to eat, that is the key to making a keto diet work, either way, this is going to involve some math, so pick your poison. Earlier in the book, a balance of 5% intake from carbohydrates, 20% from protein, and 75% from fat were mentioned. That means, if you're eating 2500 kcal a day, 5% will come from carbohydrates, around 125, 20% from protein, 500 calories, and the rest from fat, 1875. This obviously varies from person to person, if you're eating 3,000 or 2,000, the total amount of calories will change, but the percentage doesn't. This is where it's important to know how many calories you need per day - it depends on weight, body composition, gender, age, and activity level.

Another way to think about it, if you're more in mind of counting out servings, is grams of net carbohydrates. What are net carbohydrates, you might ask? Net profit is how much profit you've made after you've paid your loan shark off for your gambling debt and your investors for the labor on your getaway car, net carbs are a similar concept. Net carbs are the total carbs in your box of pasta or bag of spinach with the fiber subtracted from it. Why is the fiber subtracted? Because your body can't actually use fiber for calories, fiber works on you would use drain in a sink, to clean itself out. Regardless, what you want to aim for is 20 grams of net carbs or under, which can be increased the further into ketosis you get.

For the sake of clarity and consistency, the remainder of this book will use the percentage-based model.

How do I do this and what should I expect?

The keto diet isn't for everybody, and not everybody is willing to go crazy and try out scores of new foods just so they have enough variety not to go crazy and still keep themselves in ketosis. Like with anything else, it's always good to start slow and slowly ramp up the intensity. Don't go crazy and try mixing leaf lard into your coffee on your first day of keto. For one, that'll probably be gross and turn you off from it, and it's also a magnificent waste of good quality lard.

It's important to analyze and internalize a few things before going into this as well. Deep down, it's vital to know that fat is not the enemy. Fat in most of its forms is good for you and good for your heart, it's just eating the wrong kind and eating it with too much starch or sugar. Get used to cooking with more if it – pour a bit of extra olive oil or spoon some extra butter into the pan next time you fry a pork chop; it's good for you! Once you get used to it, it'll be hard to come off eating like that, trust me; it's delicious. It pays to be able to cook when doing keto as well, your ability to find a keto-appropriate frozen meal would probably be limited, expensive, and frustrating, and you can keep your taste buds and wallet happy. Do some research and try to modify some classic recipes that you're a fan of to a more keto appropriate version.

Use a classic human behavioral control system – in-group shaming, as a way to stick to your diet.

Inform your friends and cohorts of your new plan, and let them know that it's important that you experience a great dishonor from them if you sway from your diet. Social pressures are a huge motivating factor for a lot of people, use it to your dietary advantage! Finally, know what sort of disasters you're potentially in for. If you're skipping through this book and haven't read the previous chapter, there's a concise and informative (if I do say so myself) breakdown of the keto flu. Know what it is, how to avoid it if possible, and how to treat it.

Perhaps the best way to get into the keto diet isn't to one day start eating a half-dozen eggs and family's worth of bacon, but to slowly reduce carbohydrate intake over the course of a week or so. If you normally get 50% of your calories from carbohydrates, bring it down by 5% each day, compensating with increased fat, until you're down to 5%. And do this with foods you like – if you're partial to butter and fatty meat, eat some butter and fatty meat. If you're more of an avocado and eggs person, stick to avocado and eggs. Enjoy an extra couple of eggs and extra avocado instead of smearing it on toast. Before you know it, your body will be a veritable anti-fat furnace, and you'll be shedding pounds in no time, the key is to be patient and take it slow.

What to eat?

If you're like most people, your breakfast might consist of some kind of grain, maybe oatmeal or whole wheat cereal, with a side of protein and/or fruit, something to that effect. You're going to need to scrap this convention entirely if you want your body to enter starvation mode without actually starving. Certain foods absolutely need to be avoided 100% of the time from here on out, common staples like rice, corn, pasta, beans, and bread, many dairy products aside from butter, yogurt, and cheese, of course, sugar in all its nefarious forms.

What you can and should eat are things like healthy fats, olive, avocado, and coconut oils, butter, humanely-raised, and harvested lard and tallow. For protein, you should eat meat, poultry, eggs, seafood, cheese and plain, whole-fat Greek yogurt. Most or all of your carbs should come from non-starchy vegetables – no potatoes or corn. Think vegetables in the cabbage family, broccoli, cauliflower, kale, cabbage, and brussels sprouts are some of the healthiest things you can eat. Spinach, zucchini, and summer squash are also good choices; essentially, almost all vegetables are good as long as they're low in carbs.

Tying it together

Going keto can be an intimidating process, but as long as you set a comprehensive and well-structured goal plan for yourself, know what you're getting into and what to expect, as well as honing your cooking skills and what to eat, it doesn't have to be dietary torture. At the very worst, it can be an interesting experiment that may cause you to shed a few pounds – at best; it can be a complete shift in your lifestyle and perspective.

Chapter 5: Ketosis and How to Reach It

The metabolic process of ketosis is, obviously, the very core of the diet, the foundation from which all its principles stem from. What is its biological purpose? How exactly is it happening, and why is it so hard to reach? What is "optimal" ketosis, how does one get there, and how does one measure if one is in ketosis? All these questions and probably more than you thought you had will all be covered here, in this, the most technically involved and possibly dry chapter in this entire publication.

The purpose of ketosis

One of the interesting things about ketosis lies on the fact that it's such an obvious adaptation for the body, but still so hard to reach. The reality of all biological hardware is that it hates to expend energy. Expending energy is the exact opposite of what you're programmed to like doing, which is why getting up off the couch and going for a jog is so bloody difficult for a lot of people. Billions of years of evolution have resulted in the most complex electro-chemical structure known to science's favorite activity being loafing around and putting more energy into our systems, because who is to know when we'll need that energy to escape from a tiger or rabid gang of crocodiles. Fortunately (Or unfortunately, depending on who you ask) our day-to-day is no longer subsumed by a desperate struggle for survival, so what happens when we're putting all those calories is in we get fat and unhappy.

Many dawns past, mankind had to fight just to etch out an existence in a damp cave by a river, before agriculture, and way before firearms. Food was scarce, the only thing to eat was wild game. They would feast on their flesh, and it was speculated, especially the organ meat, for its high saturation of micronutrients, and the fat, as it provided huge amounts of energy, which made it taste great. Studies done in the 19th and 20th century of the native peoples of the arctic circle show a diet that is essentially the same, and they live just fine. The dogs eat muscle meat, and the people eat fat and organs. And then, they wouldn't eat for a day or two, so their body would start to break down all the stored fat in their systems to use as energy. When hunter-gatherers settled down to become farmers, food was aplenty, but far less rich and nutrients, and this eventually became the norm. Farming would prove to be more effective for sustaining a large population, and thus the history of humanity begins there. The purpose of ketosis is to nourish the body when food is scarce, with the original signal being from a drop in blood sugar.

Mechanism of Action

Ketosis is a complex biochemical process, and the depth of it cannot be fully covered by someone who is not working in the field of biological research, but what is done here is hopefully a more demystifying explanation than previous ones found in the book that can help you fully comprehend what's going on in your body.

When blood sugar and insulin drop low from lack of carbohydrate intake, the adipose tissue, or fat cells, of the body is triggered to release stored fatty acids to be consumed as energy. This is a simple enough principle so far, but it quickly gets hairier than a gorilla who's been using rogaine. A long chain of biochemical reactions needs to take place because fatty acids can't directly enter a cell to provide with energy. They're negatively charged, so they repel away from the positively-charged cell instead of being allowed in. What happens to fix this are fatty acids need to be transformed into the compound acetyl-CoA so our bodies can utilize them as energy. There are two paths it can go down to yield energy – we're interested in one that occurs in the liver, as the mitochondria, (essentially a cell's power plant) are most efficient at transforming them into ketones than any other cell in the body. The liver cells transform acetyl-CoA by combining two acetyl-CoA molecules to form a new one, called acetoacetyl-CoA, and then with a third acetyl-CoA molecule to yield a compound called beta-hydroxy-beta-methylglutaryl-CoA, a famous spelling test word. Another enzyme then changes this mouthful of a compound to acetoacetate, one of the three different ketone bodies. Acetoacetate can then convert, via enzyme, to a second type of ketone, beta-hydroxybutyrate. Acetoacetate and beta-hydroxybutyrate are the two types of ketones that provide energy. A third type, acetone, is also produced from the degradation of acetoacetate, and is less used for energy, and is usually the ketone detected by both those who are unfortunate enough to smell keto breath and by electronic breath readers. Acetoacetate and beta-hydroxybutyrate can then be shuttled off to various parts of the body where they are broken down into their composite pieces for fuel.

How to measure your ketosis

It is possible to easily track ketosis by a variety of different means, all of which have their ups and downs. The three available on the market are blood, breath, and urine meters. Blood is the most accurate, breath can vary based on the phase of the moon, and urine's primary use is just to tell you whether you're in ketosis. From least to most effective:

Again, primarily just used to tell you if you're in ketosis. There's not really an accurate count, counting pennies with your eyes closed is more reliable. However, if you're just getting into this new thing and are still gun shy about investing too much money, it's not a bad place to start, they're also far more ubiquitous than the other types. They're also fairly easy to use in compared to sticking yourself with a blood tester; you just hold the strip in the urine and the darker it is, the more ketones are in your urine, hypothetically. Problems with reliability lie in the fact that if you've hydrated yourself as doctors want, it'll show lighter as it dilutes the ketones. They're also known to be lighter in people who have been following the diet longer because the body is more efficient at hoovering up the ketones for energy.

The most old school breath meter in existence is, after a week or so of ketosis, trying to give your lover a peck on the mouth. If they recoil and tell you, it smells like you've been eating fruit that went bad and started hanging out with a seedy crowd, and you've been brushing your teeth and using mouthwash, you're probably in ketosis, and what's causing that smell is acetone on your breath. However, as opposed to basing your ketone count off of how much your other half recoils, other methods take advantage of modern USB technology. You plug it in and give it a blow. The downside to this is that they can run in a very high price range, in the $200 range, and they still are not as accurate as blood meters.

Blood meter:

They say you get what you pay for, and in this case, you definitely will because while you're getting the diamond standard in terms readout of your ketosis, you'll also be paying diamond prices over a period of time if you intend on keeping the diet up for any period of time. You have to pay for each strip, and they run about a buck a strip, which adds up fast. There is the chance of failed readings, but as long as you're accurate with your pricking you should be fine, but it does mean you might waste a dollar here and there. Downsides are obvious besides long-term price, and not everyone has what it takes to prick themselves in the finger.

Interpreting readings:

When you get a reading of ketone count, it'll be somewhere between 0 and 3 mmol/L.

- .5 and below doesn't count as ketosis; your body is running as normal

- .6 to 1.5 you're there, but it's light.
- 1.5 – 3.0 is your best ketosis, where you want to be to burn through the most weight.
- 3 and onward is not really necessary; it more often can indicate prolonged fasting/starvation periods than anything else. You aren't going through any more calories than those in the 1.5–3.0 range. However...
- 6 – Anything approaching this means you're getting into ketoacidosis, which can be potentially fatal. It's rare that you would reach that, but in case you do, seek medical attention immediately.

Attaining optimal ketosis

Ketosis is not a quick metabolic state to get into, as it takes your body burning through all its saved-up glucose and then it starts to break down your fatty acids. This can take up to 2 to 3 days of fasting or conscious eating on a ketogenic diet to get to. And when it begins, it's not exactly the most efficient process. It can take up to two weeks for your body to start utilizing beta-hydroxybutyrate in amounts considered strong enough to fend off the feeling of impending death from the keto flu, which is why when you enter ketosis, it's crucial to stick with it for a few days to assure that your body can adapt and take full advantage of its capability to produce energy for you.

Reaching optimal ketosis is essentially the same thing as reaching lite ketosis. It's just a manner of patience and delicate balance of nutrients.

Many parts of the body can't live off ketone bodies alone; they still require a fair bit of glucose to keep functioning, your brain most importantly. Fats are composed of fatty acids and glycerol, and while the fatty acids can be used to form ketones, the glycerol is metabolized by your liver through gluconeogenesis to form new glucose for your brain. Hearty contributions from lactate and amino acids are also to thank for producing glucose. Normally, as you undergo ketosis, your brain starts off only getting around 30% of its energy from the ketones, but as ketones meet and greet and become chummy with parts of your anatomy, that will rise to 70%, and it prefers beta-hydroxybutyrate, which, if you recall, is also the compound that helps the neurons develop more mitochondria, to deal with its increased energetic load.

Regardless, about a third of your brain will still sequester itself off and refuse to mingle with its new sources of energy, and that's where gluconeogenesis comes in. Your brain is the most selfish organ in your body and thinks of itself more highly the "lower" organs, so all the glucose you're producing from the glycerol and proteins and your small amounts of carbs are going right there. That's how your brain stays fed on keto, by stealing from the rest of your body. But remember, the wrong amount of protein and not enough fat can throw it off. This is sort of where it gets tricky. You need to get enough protein in to prevent your muscles from wasting and maintain your brain health, but not too much to throw you out of it. That's why it's so incredibly important to make sure that you're getting exactly what you need and staying stuffed with fat instead of more meat/eggs/fish.

Conclusion:

Ketosis is a complex biochemical process that comes about from a cascade of reactions with a lot of long, garbled names, and a lot of enzymes that weren't named here, but ends up in a magnificent process that can be abused for weight loss purposes. Doubtless, our hunter-gatherer ancestors never could have conceived of such a world, where food was so abundant that we had to manipulate our bodies into starving ourselves without the starvation aspect, nor a world where it was so easy to track and measure your starvation for optimal weight loss, but the future is truly a magnificent place, and with modern technology, reaching optimal ketosis for optimum weight loss is as easy as a prick of the finger.

Chapter 6: Making Keto Work for Everybody

This chapter should begin by admitting that "everybody" is a misnomer; you can't make anything work for everybody, there's always some miniscule percentage that has reasons as to why they can't. Sometimes, their simple inherent biology isn't compatible with it, or they can't stand the dietary restrictions, or because of a sport they play or their job, they need the quicker energy supplied by carbohydrates. But keto can still work for virtually everybody, provided they have the discipline and the know-how.

Keto on a budget

Reaching ketosis is a double-edged sword. Unless you're starving yourself, your diet is massively different than what you're used to, and let's be realistic here, a diet heavy in fat, high-quality oil, meat, and vegetables can add up quickly. There's a reason that we sometimes refer to the carbs and fibrous roughage on our plates as the "filler food," because it's cheap and abundant and fills you up. Whether you're a poor college kid, in between jobs or trapped at a bad gig or just a penny-pincher, it's easy to eat keto on a budget as long as you keep your head in it.

The first thing to remember is that if you're eating more fat, you're going to be less hungry inherently, so you don't have to refuel between meals or snack constantly, and hey, you might even be able to skip a meal or two. Less snacking and less time eating by itself is a money-saving strategy. You will also find that a large reason as to why we feel hungry is purely from adaptation – your stomach is accustomed to being fed whenever it wants, so it gets spoiled, when really, missing a meal won't render you an emaciated skeleton, not when you have plenty of energy stored away.

And just because you're on keto doesn't mean that you have to start buying grass-fed steak in massive qualities, just as long as you're getting enough protein, breaking the bank isn't necessary.

Tips for keeping your wallet and belly full

- First off, as a universal rule when it comes to buying groceries, consider buying in bulk. Buying in bulk is usually cheaper per pound or per ounce provided you know how to preserve your goods; it will save you many a trip to the grocery store. This especially applies to things like coconut and olive oil, you can buy a huge jug, and as long as it's capped right, it will last for months.

- Consider shopping at farmer's markets, usually the smaller, the better. Anything that has grown to resemble a state fair with a lot of cooked food vendors generally has higher prices. People are more open to bargaining, and certain in-season vegetables can come much cheaper. If you catch a deal, even meats and other animal products can be cheaper than the bigger stores, and usually better raised as well.

- Immigrant stores are similar; most of them have certain keto-friendly foods, eggs, chicken, oils, and the like marked down compared to the more "vanilla" stores.

- When looking for animal proteins, skip the steak and go for the tougher, cheaper cuts. Whole picnic hams, pork shoulder roasts, whole beef chuck roast and brisket, and whole chickens are cheaper than their broken-down forms. Chickens are easy to break down once you get the swing of it and can be cooked in bulk and frozen. Anything off the skeleton that you don't eat can be saved and boiled in a pot to make stock to use for later.

- If in-season low-carb produce is still expensive, buy it frozen. Frozen produce is still just as nutrient dense as regular produce and comes in huge bags. Avoid canned, as they're usually so hard-boiled than they manage to sap the nutrients out of them.

- If you can get past it, consider eating organ meats. This also might be a good thing to look out for at a farmer's markets. Ask your local farmer what he does with his offal, and if it's within your budget and you're feeling adventurous give it a try. Offal is oftentimes more nutritious in a lot of ways than "regular" meat, so in addition to meeting your keto goals, you'll be getting a lot of micronutrients as well.

- When it comes to offal, it helps to dip your toes in the water before going all out and buying a whole pig head or something similarly ghastly. Try making stock with pig feet, as they're filled with healthy collagen. If you can get past that, try out tongue and heart. They're essentially the same kind of muscle you're used to eating, just in a more familiar shape. Tongue is fantastic braised and heart is great seared in a pan and sliced thin. The liver has a stronger taste, but soaked in milk and cooked right can be evened out. If it's still too much, mix it in with some ground meat – pork is almost always cheaper, and ground heart is cheaper than that.

- Get familiar with cheese and eggs. Cheese is a fantastic source of protein and fat, and a little goes a long way, and eggs are cheap and very nutritious. Certain cheeses can even be cooked in a pan to form a kind of keto flatbread or cracker, with the same crunch but made from cheese.

- Finally, if you can't cook, learn how to. Know your seasonings; they're a good investment to help null the pain of repetitive meals. Find out what you like and what goes on what – for instance, what I've learned as an enthusiastic home cook is that garlic apparently goes good on everything. Eating out is expensive, even at cheap places, and oftentimes they won't be able to account for your diet. If you can throw together a good keto meal from chicken livers, a can of tomatoes, garlic, and a half cup of coconut oil, you're probably about three steps ahead of most people.

Keto and the holidays

I know it's the holidays because I can feel every cell in my gastrointestinal system screaming for mercy from the nuclear carbohydrate bomb I've forced dropped on it. Something about the holidays really gets people eating like crap – the cold weather, the abundance of food, the sense of comfort and security from being around your family. These factors all combine into a nightmarish wraith that will chase you down (mentally) stuffing cookies and pasta and panettone down your throat and won't rest until a couple of notches has loosened your belt loop. Fear not – for there are ways to banish this wraith back to the sugary hell from whence he came.

The first and foremost thing to remember is self-control. Unless you are running the entire holiday show and making ALL THE FOOD, you can't control what your friends and family will bring, but you can control what you actually put in your piehole. Grandma will probably not change her 400-year-old Bavarian pastry recipe because the grandkid whose name she can't remember is following some strange new diet. Keep in mind why you're following this diet, keep your goals in mind, and what step you're on to reach them. You are in charge of you. Only you can make you eat that cookie or hunk of bread. It's a thousand times easier not to eat something than to endeavor to burn it off later.

Center your activities around things besides eating. As a culture, I think it's collectively fine to admit that the food is half the reason we are all still at peace during the holidays. It keeps us happy and sedated and makes our great aunt's rambles about the depression a little easier to sit through. But there are other activities – talk to your family, help them cook so you can sneak in your own creations. Play a ball game, go caroling, pumpkin carving, pumpkin throwing, volunteer in a soup kitchen, something that doesn't revolve around food.

When it comes to the table though, bring something that is in the clear for your gut. Roasted green vegetables or a salad, bring a meat dish, something that you know you can come back to if the turkey is double-breaded and the only side is candied yams. Realistically, they won't be like that and take advantage of the wealth of food around you. Good chance that somewhere around the dinner table there's something that fits your diet pick and choose the meat and green vegetables.

It's also important to know where carbs could be lurking in ambush - gravy is basically an emulsion of the best things in life – fat, flour, and meat broth, but the flour kicks you out of your diet. If the turkey is drier than the desert, opt for the dark meat, always richer in taste, micronutrients, and fat. You can even try making a ketogenic version of a holiday classic if you feel like flexing your ability and showing off your flashy new diet to your old relatives who still communicate via telegram.

Finally, if your resolve breaks and you start reaching for the rolls and rice, stick to those closest to your heart, (Your gut?) so you can truly appreciate it. Set a limit ahead of time, but while you're eating it, savor it, because both of us know this is the last you'll get for a while.

Keto and going out

Everyone likes a night on the town, but how do you properly impress your date with your nutritional awareness and stick to your diet? Is it possible to stick to keto and still embarrass yourself on the dance floor after a bit too much alcohol? This section aims to answer these questions.

What do I order?

Obviously, avoid the complimentary bread, skip out on the pasta, and don't eat dessert. But there is more finesse to it – many restaurants will let you replace your starch with a side vegetable or salad instead, so keep your eyes open for that option. If you're a hip enough burger joint, you can get it wrapped in lettuce like a little burgerrito hybrid. If you can't avoid the starch with your meal, try forcing it on your friend, or simply not eating it and tossing it in the trash, so the temptation isn't there.

Many places, sandwich joints in particular, usually offer a salad with a protein instead of a bread. Opt for that instead, and add extra fat where you can. Ask for a splash of olive oil on your steamed veggies, or an extra serving of dressing for your salad. Remember to ask the waiter about the nutritional content of anything not properly explained, finding extra sugars in salad dressings is very common. If they don't have a proper healthy dressing, simply ask for olive oil and vinegar. Always drink water or unsweet tea or coffee with your meals.

Alcohol

Alcohol is a whole different ball game. Beer and wine both are filled with carbs, so those are right out, and if you're partial to living in the moment with sugary cocktails despite the hangover they give, I have bad news for you. You'll have to resort to only drinking hard liquor and water to get the courage to ask the girl/guy on the sidelines out, anything else doesn't fit. Certain cocktails might fit, drinks with pickle or olive brine are in the clear, but generally, if it tastes good, spit it out. There is an upside, as a night of all spirits and water is possibly the "cleanest" most efficient and cost-effective way to get drunk, even if it's not pleasant. On the downside, it's all too real a fact that alcohol lowers inhibitions, so be careful not to have too much and drink responsibly.

It's perfectly possible to maintain your diet while globetrotting, but knowing the background of where you're going is vital. Some countries and locations follow a diet with a higher carbohydrate count than others, and it's important to get informed and find out alternatives before you go. The same principles apply as when going out, just on a larger scale. If your vacation is more active, hiking the Appalachian trail, you're going to need energy. Make sure to keep this in mind when packing your trail food. The perfect food for this sort of activity would be pemmican, a native American trail food made of dried meat and fat. If you can't find it or make it, many stores sell salami and other cured meats. Cured and smoked meats are not the best foods for you, but the kinds that preserved more traditionally tend to have less of a damaging effect, and it keeps you in ketosis and not starving, which is the most important thing.

Keto is a powerful weight loss tool that, with some knowledge and discipline, can work for those of us on a budget, going out, traveling, and during the holidays. It's not easy – but doing something worth it rarely is, but it's easily possible once you apply what you learned in this chapter.

Chapter 7: Is Keto a Good Fit for You?

In the last chapter, we talked about how ketosis can potentially work for everybody, but that doesn't necessarily mean it's the best diet for *everybody*. This chapter encourages you to reflect on your lifestyle, in all its facets, to see if this new trendy diet will fit you. All the pieces that define who you are – your current diet, occupation, your ethnic and religious background, where and who you live with, personality, social relations, and activity level provide you with the answer to the question "is this is the right diet for me?"

One thing to keep in mind is that if you're interested in the diet and are confident you can reach ketosis, try it out. See how you feel, see if you think it can be a viable option, provided everything else in your life is in alignment. You won't know until you try, you might get on the diet and lose the weight you've been trying to lose for the last year and feel great and energized. If by some chance, you fall off the wagon and the issue wasn't you're your willpower, no harm done, you tried it, and factors outside your control means it didn't work for you. That's how things happen sometimes.

This is the most important factor of all, knowing yourself and your behaviors. If you know, you're the kind of person who can't resist a cookie or just loves pasta to an unhealthy degree, start rethinking your dieting options. Even lacking a detail-oriented personality can put you in a bind, as it's a very sensitive diet. Let's re-establish this now - keto is not for all types of people, simply because it requires a lot more conscious decision making and planning than what we're used to when it comes to food. Not everyone is like that, and that's okay. Calculating a percentage of fat, protein, and calories to eat everyday and then revamping your eating habits around them isn't exactly rocket science, but it's still a hassle for most of us. If you have problems resisting temptation, or if food is a comfort and a passion for you, or the way you pay your bills, these can all conflict. And it helps to be experienced in dieting – if you've counted calories before, if you've gone on a prolonged fast, or if simply nothing else has worked for you, and you're getting desperate, you might excel on this diet.

Regimented people who are more interested in form and results than taste probably will end up doing better on this diet as well. Openness is one of the "big five" personality traits, and more open people are always interested in trying new things. If you're a very open person who likes variety, what boils down to cutting yourself off from an entire food group and pigeonholing you into a small window would quickly drive you up a wall from monotony and cause you to break your diet.

Current diet

How you eat right now is important, which is why, if you're interested in ketosis, it's important to ask yourself why you want to go on it. If your current diet works for you and you're living with no problems, weight or otherwise, why try to change it? Curiosity is certainly a factor, and by all means, try it if you want, but don't try to force it if it doesn't work like you thought. If you need to have your meals with a glass of oil instead of water, there's a red flag.

If you're interested in the diet but don't need all health benefits it can yield, it could be a better idea to try out a "lite" version of it, the low-carb diet, or try fasting. The low-carb diet will yield the same sensation of fullness as keto that leads to fewer calories consumed. Fasting is an excellent technique for weight management, changing your relationship with food, building self-control, has the benefit of spiking growth hormone, known for its anti-aging properties. But, at the end of the day, if your current diet is chock full of carbs and you're living just fine, it might not be worth it to go into ketosis.

If you're a football player, fighter, rugby player, or any athlete whose sport is based on anaerobic systems of producing energy, you should rethink your decision. You're going to need a lot of carbohydrates going into those muscles to keep everything functioning as best it possibly can. If you're working out hard in high-intensity intervals several days a week, being on ketosis can make you feel like you're circling the drain. But if you're a runner who's putting in 6 miles a day, this could be the perfect fit. Even people who walk a lot, for work or pleasure, can make good use of ketosis. Weight training lies somewhere in between a properly adapted weightlifter might feel fine on ketosis or even fasted and be able to pull like they always do. The issue is if you were interested in starting off weightlifting and tried doing it during keto, the proper physiological adaptations would not have occurred, and you wouldn't be able to perform anywhere near your best.

Eating keto, even if you're doing it on a budget, can get expensive, especially if you want to indulge in something besides organ meat and drinking a cup of

oil every now and then. Certain parts of the country –
and certain parts of the world, of course, may have
extremely inflated food prices or simply poor access
to ketogenic foods. If you're living in a more rural
area of an underdeveloped country, most of the
options for food are probably starchy, as they're the
easiest to grow in mass. It may be possible to eat a
ketogenic diet, but it may not be worth the trouble
and extra time investment, or you may not be able to
get your macronutrient balance right every day. Other
places may be "food deserts" where access to fresh
and unprocessed is very limited or impossible. While
eating keto may be possible on a diet of slim jims and
hotdogs, it's not healthy or affordable.

If you have housemates who drink often or eat
your food (hopefully, buddies of yours), maybe you
live a bit more "communally" than the average
home, that would also be a problem. Peer pressure is
a very real and very effective phenomenon. Having
social pressures every single day can quickly wear
down even the most resolved dieter. Or they may
sometimes eat your food, but in return, offer you a
slice of their pizza - something to that effect - and
you figure some food is better than no food, right? In
addition, snacks or alcohol laying around everywhere
can be a temptation that you don't need. On the flip
side, living with your parents can also make it a

challenge unless you're willing to take matters of cooking into your own hands. Coming home to a comforting home-cooked meal every day is an alluring pull, not even counting on the advanced form of social pressures parents can use.

Type of employment

Different types of jobs have different caloric needs and stress levels, and stress affects eating. Not to disparage any career choices, but jobs like doctor, nurse, heavy equipment operator are generally more stressful than a receptionist or a writer. A lot of people stress eat, and a lot of people are stressed out because of their job, and stress eating often leads to poorly thought out choices. Amount of physical exertion at work is a factor as well. Consider the manual laborer, he or she might be performing the same kind and level of activity as an athlete, the kind of person who moves bricks all day or swings a sledgehammer will need an energy source that can provide for these big, powerful movements. Meanwhile, someone who sits a chair for four to five hours at a time will need fewer calories and can probably perform fine just breaking down their own fat. In fact, the ketogenic diet would probably greatly aid someone like that as sitting has been linked to high mortality, probably via the accumulation of excess weight.

Some of the most powerful cables in the world that bind us come from our families. They're the cradle of our personality. They fostered us, it gives us a context as to where we came from so we can know where we're going and get the impression that we're a part of something bigger than ourselves. In a more practical sense, the foods we eat are massively affected by how we grew up and what we can cook competently, or at least, make not taste like death. Even if you don't live with or around your family anymore, the imprints they made are as fissures in you, massive and unavoidable. Someone from India would be more predisposed to following a vegan or vegetarian diet, chocked full of naan bread and lentils. An Italian would have been eating pasta and pizza since he was a boy. Sometimes it's just hard to make the jump into a new diet where you're not confident that you'll be able to feed yourself without wanting to vomit up three times the amount of oil you're used to consuming at once.

Religion is also a factor for a lot of people. As the genesis of society itself lies in grain farming since time immemorial bread has been intrinsic to religious rituals. This is observed in almost every mass organized religion worldwide. Imagine how awkward it would be to tell your priest that you can't take communion because you're doing keto? Many religions have strict rules about what you can eat and when, and if you're a true devout this can be problematic as you must choose between spirituality and diet. If there can be no compromise brokered, that would be a problem moving ahead. The only alternative would be to create your own religion centered around the keto diet, which probably would have some kind of root in primitive mysticism and animism that would necessitate shamanic trances, which is a whole different can of worms.

Social life

The final thing to be considered is your gang of miscreants you chum around with. Would they be supportive, or would they chide you about your new diet and actively discourage you? Would they take it a step further, and actively dump sugar onto what you're eating without telling you, and sneak breadcrumbs into food they said with keto? For starters, if you have friends like that, they probably are not very good friends, and you should consider getting new ones. But if your friends are actually normal and the worst they do is tease you about it, it could be worth it to have a talk with them and let them know that you're trying to improve yourself, and if they're worth their salt, they'll understand and desist. However, if you are all a bunch of raving party animals and going out on the town is a common occurrence, this could also lead to trouble. As alluded to earlier, drinking will lower inhibitions. In addition to just being plain not very good for you overall, if you have many bouts of drinking over the course of a month, there's a realistic chance that might break your diet at some point. Think about your habits, your friend's habits, because they will affect you, and consider whether keeping your relationship as it is might sabotage your diet. The best solution would be adaptation on their end and your end, with both working to making you happy, but obviously, this can't always happen.

So, is it realistic for you?

Once you consider these factors, everything from family to personality, social life to activity, you'll be properly equipped to know if this is the move for you. There's no perfect diet for everyone, and everyone is different. If you decide to try out the keto diet and find that it's not for you, there's no harm in going back to the drawing board and trying out something new to see if it will get the results you're looking for, just don't be too hard on yourself and try to sustain something unsustainable. Remember to really ruminate on these factors, because while you may be a lapsed Catholic jogger who works in an office, and that really seems like a good fit for someone going on a diet, if you're used to shotgunning beers with your boys on the weekends, your liver will be too occupied cleaning you out to make ketones.

Chapter 8: Exercise and Keto

Ketosis and exercise may initially seem like a poor combination. Exercise, by necessity, requires a lot of carbohydrates for energy, right? Well, not exactly. Scores of professional athletes have had great results on ketosis, and it's true that they're genetically blessed, have a ridiculous work ethic, and the best coaches, dieticians, and doctors money can buy, but with the right head on your shoulders, there's no reason why you can't excel on the field or in the weight room while keeping the fat-burning engine lit. There's a real downside that's been alluded to previously, and it's that unfortunately, ketosis and high-intensity training don't mix, because no matter what you do, it's powered by glycogen, which is made from carbohydrates, or at least not traditional ketosis, with a modified plan, results can be had. There are still plenty of other modalities to follow, though. Supplementation should also be rethought, as the change in your macronutrient profile will doubtless change what you need and what you don't need.

A few considerations

To really understand what this chapter is going to dive in to, a basic understanding of your body's energy systems is needed. To keep it short and sweet (or short and fatty, I guess) your body has three main energy systems for exercise. Ketosis really does good for one of them.

From shortest to longest duration of activity, there is the phosphagen system, the anaerobic system, and the aerobic system. The phosphagen system is used for heavy weightlifting - it's for very short, powerful movements. This isn't affected by ketosis because it's neither glucose fed nor fat fed, it's something else entirely. A good way to remember how the phosphagen system works is by thinking of it as any very powerful movements that last under 10-12 seconds. In other words, it's irrelevant and if you happen to be a world class powerlifter/golfer you can go on keto and survive the workout.

The anaerobic system is used for 10 seconds to up to a minute or more, depending on the athlete, of all-out maximum effort activity like wrestling, boxing, team sports, the more "sporty" sorts of sports. This system gets hit the hardest by ketosis, and while you probably can go keto and do some of this, you're going to feel like Jacob wrestling God in the desert after. This is potentially doable, but there's a good chance of reduced performance, and you may have to tweak your diet a fair bit to get it to work, this will be covered later on.

The final system is aerobic, which after a few minutes starts knocking on the door to your fat cells to ask for donations to its starving muscle tissue. It burns through the stored up glucose in your muscles, but nowhere near to the degree that anaerobic activity does. This system is least affected by ketosis it's functioning fairly similarly to how your body works naturally anyway.

Remember that going into ketosis takes time, and at first, you may feel less like a sleek fat-eating machine and more like a person covered in grease who can't think straight. This will resolve – eventually, your body will adapt, and you will find a way to wash the butter from your last meal off your hands. It's good to wait until you feel back to your old self again before trying to do your run or pull your usual deadlift, which shouldn't be too hard as my motivation to crush weight and cross-country run is dampened when I feel like my brain has been transformed into concrete.

Once you feel like you can walk across the room without getting lost, don't go nuts, keep your workouts familiar. Physiological adaptations happen over time to the body to be good at a certain physical skill; tendons strengthen, muscle cross-sectional area increases, the heart, and lungs get more powerful, your body knows what it's doing. But if you try to get into ballistic cross country skiing instead of your usual round in the weight room, things may not end up so pretty. In addition, if you change too much at once, regardless if you succeed or fail, there are too many variables at play to tell you why and how it worked or didn't work.

Make sure your calories are where they need to be. Keto is notorious (or famous, more positively) for keeping appetite down, which is great if you're going to be watching TV all day or playing solitaire while pretending to be working, but not so great if you're trying to swim the English Channel. If you're going to be exercising you really need those calories and all your fat. So chow down on that last bag of pork rinds before the race, you'll need it.

How to change your body composition

For a lot of people, shedding fat is the primary objective of exercise. Well, that's great news, because the ketogenic diet is designed for that, and double powerful when combined with exercise. As you know, when performing bouts of aerobic exercise, glycogen is partially bypassed in favor of delicious fatty ketones, meaning that when you exercise in ketosis, you're really speeding up that autophagy of fatty tissue during and after exercise.

Weightlifters, bodybuilders, and any number of other athletes often have to change weight classes for a meet or show. For putting on weight, aim to eat an additional 300 calories a day from fat. The inverse is the same – for losing weight, drop 300 to 500 calories a day, from both dieting and exercise.

It is still *extremely* important to eat enough protein as if you don't, your body will go delusional from lack of carbohydrates and start seeing your muscle as a sugary treat, almost identically to how cartoon characters would see each other as ice-cream sundaes when trapped on a desert island. A good metric to go by for those athletes looking to pack on muscle is **one gram per pound of bodyweigh**t, enough to keep your muscle from wasting away and keep you growing. Usually, I recommend figuring out your protein requirements first and basing the rest of your daily nutrition around that. However many grams protein you eat will be that 20% or of your daily intake, and thus fat and carbohydrates are adjusted for it.

To give you a live demonstration of how to eat to try to pack on muscle; on a 2,000 calorie diet, if you're eating 100 grams of protein a day, which is 400 calories, and 20% of your daily calories, you'd need to eat an additional 166 grams of fat, about 1500 calories. The last 100 calories should come from carbs to fill in the last 5%, 25 grams.

Note that this is most likely not enough for the average bodybuilder to put on weight, but is merely meant to show you how to properly structure your diet when you're trying to pack on muscle.

If doing both keto and continuing to wrestle is unavoidable, consider how you're going to eat. One modification of the ketogenic diet is called the targeted ketogenic diet and it - now don't spit out your steak - briefly throws you out of ketosis for the purposes of exercise performance. Your muscles need that quick-acting fuel to be able to contract right, right? Right! But if you time it, so you're eating anywhere from 25 to 50 grams of carbs, a light to moderate amount, before you work out, along with some protein, anywhere from an hour to half an hour beforehand, it should give you the boost you need to not feel like an Egyptian slave building the pyramids. It's actually beneficial if you want to keep your muscle quality as high as possible if you're doing this as well because your old buddy insulin comes out of his den to move glucose into the cells, and he also has the added benefit of slowing muscle degradation during your workout.

For the really dedicated amongst us, it helps even to know what kind of sugar to eat. Dextrose and glucose are the ones that are taken in an express train right to your muscles, usually found in candy than in fruit, so it's an excuse to eat that piece of candy you found under your car seat a week ago. If you want to be really precise, glucose gel packets are also available, or some kind of sugary sports drink works as well because they also contain electrolytes which you're going to be going through at a fast during exercise.

Finally, it's a good idea always to have a good amount of protein after a workout, as that is when your body's sensitivity to it is highest, and you need it the most to fuel your muscular restructuring and prevent any breakdown of existing muscle tissue.

You may be wondering if knocking yourself out of ketosis will mean you have a hard time getting back in. The short answer is no, as long as you follow the diet after your workout you'll be getting your ketone count back up in no time, provided you didn't eat too many carbs in the first place. The longer answer is still no, but there are things you can do to mitigate your brief visit with the old you. Steady-state mild cardio, maybe a fast walk or slow jog, has been shown to lower insulin levels. Have a refreshing chug of MCT, medium-chain triglyceride oil, sometime before, during, or after your workout, as MCTs are repurposed into ketones in no time. The reality of all this is that it is largely irrelevant, as long as you follow the diet you'll go back into ketosis just fine, and there are a bunch of different factors to see if you even left it in the first place. How hard and long you worked out will change it, probably putting you back in if you burned through your carby treat, and how long you've been in ketosis in the first place matter a lot.

Ketosis and weightlifting

For the average joes, it's important to know which training style yours mostly resembles and work from there. A ketogenic diet can work in harmony with weightlifting, but it depends on what kind of weightlifting you're doing and the twisting of a few factors.

Different schools of movement

As easy as it would be to say "ketosis and weight lifting" are compatible or not compatible, it is unfortunately not so cut and dry. For starters "weightlifting" is something of deceiving term, as it can vary depending on the athlete. In a strict sense, "weightlifting" refers to Olympic weightlifting, a sport centered around two major lifts and accessory movements to those lifts. Olympic weightlifting's two lifts are the clean and jerk and the snatch. Olympic weightlifting is a high-skill sport, with both lifts requiring exceptional balance and mobility, not to mention loads of explosive power. In general, it uses the phosphagen system the most.

Another common type of training is powerlifting, which is centered around three lifts, the bench press, squat, and deadlift. Powerlifting is less technically demanding and less explosive (Powerlifting still requires tons of explosive strength, but the movements are by nature never as dynamic or quick as Olympic movements.) but rewards brutal, slow strength, and also makes great use of the phosphagen system, doubtless with bleed in from the glycogen-fed anaerobic system.

Bodybuilding also falls under the umbrella of "weightlifting," and Arnold Schwarzenegger doing bicep curls in a state of ecstasy is probably what most non-athletes picture when the word "weightlifting" is said. Unlike powerlifting and Olympic lifting, bodybuilding is not about how high your total with two or three exercises is. Bodybuilding is about trying to get your muscles as big as possible, which bodybuilding is a far more open training style than Olympic lifting or powerlifting. Training is more focused on set ranges of repetition and rest times that are designed to maximize muscular hypertrophy - the size of the muscle. To achieve this, bodybuilding needs to maximize time under tension. To water down years of scientific research to an easy-to-remember maxim, the more time under tension - the time your bicep is contracted while curling a weight - the bigger they get. Bodybuilders manipulate their physiology by using moderate weight with higher-repetition sets and a short rest time to maximize their muscle growth by maximizing how long they're contracted for. This range can be where from 8 to 12 reps, with rest times lasting anywhere from 30 seconds to two minutes and weight anywhere from 50% to 75%. There may be some commonalities amongst bodybuilder programming, but they tend to vary person to person more so than powerlifting or Olympic lifting would. Because of the nature of having to get every muscle in the body as large and symmetrical as possible, bodybuilding training times might run longer than powerlifting or Olympic lifting. Bodybuilding will use the phosphagen system for its heavier lifting, and for its burnout muscle-stressing movements, will make more use of the anaerobic system.

With all this in mind, for the average dieter and weight enthusiast, it's doubtful that they strictly train like any of these athletes, which is where things get hairier. Each of these training styles stresses a different energy system more than the other, with bodybuilding probably doing the best job at depleting muscle glycogen and Olympic lifting relying the most on the phosphagen system and powerlifting hanging out in the middle. It's important to know how you're going to train. Doing high repetition exercises would fall under the glucose-fed system, things like 8–12 reps, and when your muscle glycogen is low, your results will suffer.

How do I apply this?

Now that we have an idea of what kinds of lifting are out there, we can think about our goal. If you're looking to develop a lot of power and strength, usually with rep ranges in the 1 to 5 range, the domain of Olympic lifting and powerlifting, and you've already adapted to your new diet, you can safely assume that you'll be able to keep working out unhindered.

If your style is more bodybuilding or mixed style, with a lot of variations in things like exercises from day to day and rep ranges and rest times and a longer workout, you might feel like you're being put through a strange form of self-induced torture. Your body is going to need extra glycogen, because every time you do a set of high-rep bicep curls or lunges, your body starts tapping into its glycogen-fed system, which you have depleted because of your diet. If you want to excel and your workout has a bunch of these high-rep movements, consider eating your carbs before you work out to give yourself the energy to keep yourself from passing out on a strenuous lift.

It should be noted that all training types use all energy systems to some degree. It could be said, for example, that 80% of Olympic-style training uses creatine phosphate for fuel, but physiology is never that cut, and dry and inevitably other systems will be used to smaller degrees. For example - many programs based around developing power usually have a fair amount of "bodybuilding-style" accessory work to assure that all the helping muscles in the lift are also up to top shape, and oftentimes these rep ranges can exceed the usual for 1 to 5 reps power and thus expire the creatine phosphate-fed system and start tapping into the glycogen system. If this has been happening to you, remember your body talks to you, and if you're suffering through your power-focused workout, you should consider following the targeted ketogenic diet and supplement with carbs 30 minutes to an hour before your workouts.

Ketosis and cardio

Ketosis and cardio really are a fantastic couple and have been bedmates maybe even going back to before recorded history. As a quick aside, consider what might have been the human condition throughout history, and even exists today in parts of the world. We are weaker and smaller than many animals, but some reason we still derive a lot of nutrients from their flesh. We are smart and well-adapted for endurance running, though our pace is slow, we could usually run megafauna to exhaustion. Our bodies can take that stored fat and toss it right in our furnace to keep our legs pumping so that one day, we might wipe the mammoth scourge off the face of the planet. Nothing has changed nowadays, we're still great at it, but we're much lazier and would rather just shoot it.

Activities that count as cardio would be triathlete's events, jogging, cycling, swimming, rowing, the elliptical, and dance classes. Nothing that winds you and makes you want to throw up, essentially.

If you primarily exercise by doing steady-state, unchanging submaximal cardio, defined as getting you to within 50-70% of your maximum heart rate, ketosis fits in a whole lot easier with many less dietary shenanigans than weightlifting. What's my maximum heart rate, you may ask? The shorthand for it is generally 220 minus your age. Once again, nothing is set in stone as everyone's physiology is different, but that's a good ballpark marker to go for. So if you're 27, it would be anywhere from 97 to 135 beats per minute.

If you're already a cardio athlete, once you've adapted, you're good to go. But still, take things slow. Lower your intensity than what you're used to and work your way back up. Intensity, for cardio, is defined as your heart rate. If you're a carbohydrate-fed cardio athlete, who has gamed their heart rate to be able to operate at 70%, drop it down to 60% or 50% and try to make it your usual time. If you feel good, great; you've successfully managed to make the jump. If not, don't get discouraged. Wait a few more days and try it again, your body might need more time to flood fatty acids into your bloodstream.

If you're new to cardio and keto, and which case, you're probably looking to lose a lot of weight, congratulations on taking the first steps, and when you inevitably feel like there's an invisible metabolic vampire sapping you of energy after your first keto-fed session on a treadmill, the pain does abate. It takes a few weeks for a regularly-fed person to get adapted to pushing themselves for miles, so you're in for a doozy of an adaptation period. Keep your eye on the prize, and don't push yourself too far too fast or you'll get discouraged. When first beginning, try to get your heart rate at half your maximum and maintain your activity for only about 20 minutes. If you feel any joint pain, that's a sure sign to slow down. Remember that proper form is extremely important with any athletic movement, not just weightlifting, so really set those patterns of movement in your head to avoid injury and be on the path to look and feel your best.

Keto and supplementation

Any athlete worth his salt will tell you that half the fun of being active is the freedom to experiment on yourself like a mad scientist with all manner bizarre supplements, from creatine to the 57 varieties of protein powder in all of its artificial-tasting flavors. People on the keto diet may be in need of a few supplements to stay in good health, and it's important to know which common workout supplements it conflicts with and any adjustments you can make to keep taking it.

For staying healthy

This section should be proceeded with the disclaimer that supplements are not essential; that's why they're called supplements. Supplements should only be used when you need them, which, admittedly, can be hard to tell when. Keeping that in mind, some are "more" essential than others; almost all of us could use more omega-3s in our diet, for instance, and there's a good chance anyone on keto will need some electrolytes. It's perfectly possible to go on a keto diet and take no outside supplementation; it just requires an attention to detail above and beyond the usual.

- **Electrolytes**; potassium, sodium, and magnesium: Being low in any of these can make you feel like a dead man walking, and are indirectly the cause of many of the most awful keto flu symptoms - general irritation, insomnia, and muscle cramps and spasm. A little side effect of ketosis in its opening stages that a lot of people don't realize is your kidneys will be flushing you of water because of the lack of carbs, making you lose a lot of these salts in the process.

Sodium is important for proper firing of nerves and contracting of muscles. It's pretty easy to supplement this, literally just add salt to your foods. If your blood pressure is a problem, make sure not to overdo it and keep an eye on it in relation to your salt consumption.

Potassium: The first thing to know about potassium supplementation is this: Don't do it. Potassium can bleed over from the "Helps you stay alive" to "helps you stay dead" very quickly. The second thing to know is why you need it; it keeps your muscles from cramping, keeps your blood pressure steady, and is absolutely vital to keeping your heart pumping. Foods high in potassium are nuts, wild fish, and spinach, brussels sprouts, and avocado.

Magnesium: How do you figure you might be deficient in magnesium? Well, if you exist in America, that might a risk factor, as half of us are deficient. You'll also know if you have muscle cramps and spasms and problems sleeping. Men and women need anywhere from between 200 to 400 mg a day.

Calcium: Vital for muscle contractions which are necessary for everything. You'll need about 1,000 mg a day, and you can find it easily in things like whole canned fish fillets (bones and all!), yogurt and cheese, or supplementation.

◼ **Vitamin D:** One of the reasons vitamin D is important is that without it, calcium can't be absorbed, which can lead to further effects down the road in terms of muscular issues like weakness and fatigue. In addition, it's also vital for testosterone production. A good, cheap source is found right alongside calcium in canned bone-in sardines and for the more bourgeoisie amongst us (Or those who don't want sardine breath) fatty fresh fish.

◼ **Medium-Chain Triglyceride Oil, or MCT Oil**: MCT oil can function as what amounts to a cheat code for ketogenic dieters. They're immediately broken down into and shoved into the bloodstream where they can be used as ketones, and are a tasteless liquid fat that you can dump on everything you eat to make you feel full and keep you in ketosis.

- ☒ **Omega-3 Fatty Acids/Fish Oil:** There's been a lot of hubbub revolving around omega-3s in the last few years. They've been linked to improved brain health, cleansing of the arteries with lower triglyceride and higher HDL count, and reducing joint inflammation. It's fairly cheap for a giant container of them, but there are often questions about the quality of it and the potential for things like mercury or denatured acids so consider splurging. There's also some research suggesting it may be easier to absorb omega-3s in food forms, especially fish. If you don't want to break the bank and love sardines (we keep coming back to them don't we?) and fatty fish, they're a delicious, cheap, (In the case of sardines, anyway) and reliable way to get them in your diet.

- ☒ **Digestive enzymes:** Here's a strange-sounding one, but bear with me. When eating a diet higher in fat and protein than they're used to, it's not unusual that people can report some gastric symptoms and might need a little outside help until they're adapted, so they don't experience those feelings we all know and love; bloating, nausea, and vomiting. Supplemental digestive enzymes can help with these symptoms as they're literally the things your body makes to digest food but in pill form.

- ☒ **Exogenous ketones**: Ketones made outside the body, as the name suggests. They can help you stay in ketosis if you haven't measured your carb intake correctly, and potentially even induce a state of deeper ketosis. The best exogenous ketones are made from the best, most efficient endogenous ketones - look for a variety composed mostly of beta-hydroxybutyrate.

- ☒ **Green Powder**: Something I wish was an option when I was a kid. Dried, powdered greens, maybe the same kind of stuff they use to turn the spinach pasta green. But it's the perfect supplement who can't seem to jam in enough vegetables to their diet, which isn't surprising given their main macronutrient composition is carbohydrates.

Common workout supplements and keto

Athletes take all manner of interesting-sounding lab creations to get in shape, from creatine to BCAAs to whey powder. Do they mesh with keto? Some do, some don't. When picking a workout supplement, avoid the ones with added sugar, this mostly applies to pre-workout drinks and protein powders. While the science of the dangers of artificial sweeteners is up in the air, it's generally a good idea to forsake those too when you can. There are so many supplements that they can't all be covered here, especially the illegal ones, but a good rule of thumb is that if there's no sugar, you're good to go.

- **BCAAs** – Branched-chain amino acids. Not really necessary, as long as you eat enough protein. Most people who go on keto end up eating more protein anyway, so this shouldn't be necessary, but doesn't necessarily harm you.

- **Protein** – Pea, collagen, soy, whey protein, there are a million varieties, and they all have minute differences. Protein supplements work fine with keto as long as you're keeping your fat in higher percentages, and there's little to no added sugar.

- **Creatine** – One of the more infamous supplements in the world of athletics, despite it being possibly one of the most effective. Creatine supplements are used to power the creatine phosphate system, and there are serious links between its usage and improved athletic ability. Creatine and ketosis get along fine and share tea like civilized people as long as creatine contains no added sugar.

- ☒ **Taurine** - Taurine has come on to the stage in recent years because of its ability to patch a hole in ketosis' weakest point, energy system wise. It's been shown to improve anaerobic ability and reduce fatigue. Taurine has a stamp of approval for ketosis as well because it's great for what ketosis is bad at and contains no carbs.

- ☒ **Caffeine** - Caffeine is a double-edged sword on ketosis. It can raise cortisol levels, which is bad for ketosis. But, at the same time, it's fantastic for suppressing appetite, especially when blended with some coconut oil or butter, making a useful tool for weight loss. Also, there have been real, demonstrable effects that show that caffeine improves cardiovascular endurance. Whether or not caffeine is right for you is a personal question, many people can't function without it, and the increased cortisol levels aren't a problem. In fact, one of the infamous keto trends that have bled into wider society is "bulletproof coffee," the aforementioned coffee and butter, coffee and coconut oil, or for the truly daring, coffee and lard.

- ☒ **L-Citrulline** - Coming from the Latin word for "watermelon," citrulline helps promote blood flow in the body by way of obnoxiously complex biochemistry. It can lead to better pumps for bodybuilders as well as increased aerobic and anaerobic performance and would be ideal for the bodybuilder still adapting to his new diet.

Keto and exercise: A lot to consider

Exercise takes everything you know about resting metabolic rate and effectively makes it 5 times more complicated, displayed neatly by the length of this chapter. It's really impossible to know if ketosis and exercise walk hand-in-hand sweetly without knowing a lot more about exercise physiology and the types of activities themselves, which this chapter set out to illuminate. Hopefully, with this chapter ingrained into the mind and a fair bit of rumination on gripping topics like the phosphagen energy system, steady state cardio, and what supplements to take to avoid dropping like a fly after a workout, the right decision for your particular exercise wants and needs can be made.

Chapter 9: Keto While Vegan

Ketosis and a vegan diet is a tricky balancing act that is not accomplished by merely drinking coconut oil and crying. Vegan diets, as a refresher, are a diet free of all animal products, no meat, fish, eggs, dairy, or honey. They can be challenging to stick to on their own, much less trying to accomplish on keto, given that animal products tend to be more rich in fat and protein. Alas, it's not an entirely insurmountable task with enough nutritional knowledge and a fair bit of cooking tricks and tips.

For a vegan to go keto and keep their constitution, it's important that they know their healthiest options for fat and protein. Generally speaking, avocados, MCT oil, coconuts and coconut oil, fatty tofu (A thing I didn't know existed until I did my research for this chapter) and possibly the vegan's most powerful ally, nutritional yeast, especially the kind fortified with B12, will be your best friends. A keto vegan diet isn't going to be vastly different in terms of nutrient content than a regular keto diet, just very restrictive with what you can eat.

Cover your bases

Protein

Hopefully, dear reader, you are prepared for another long ramble on biochemistry, as without the knowledge you'd be scratching your head wondering why a vegan can't just eat 100 grams of seitan (extracted wheat gluten; also technically the "most" protein dense food) and call it a day. Well, the reason is because of amino acids. They are what makes up the delicious protein in all living things, and there are 20 of them. Eleven of these acids the body can make on its own, but there are nine it can't, which we need to get from food. All animal products containing protein have all nine in them wrapped up in a neat little bow, but not all plants do. In fact, there is a serious dearth of plant products that contain all nine amino acids we need, but thankfully this can be remedied by eating two kinds of plant protein together. The classic example is beans and rice, which has probably kept more people healthy than all medicine in all time ever.

Unfortunately, when going on a ketogenic diet, beans and rice aren't really an option, because while they combine to make a complete protein that the body can use for muscle growth and maintenance, they also contain a much higher percentage of carbohydrates, far too much to go ketogenic on. There are complete sources of protein, such as quinoa and buckwheat are personal favorites. The problem here is twofold; neither are super common in the western diet, so it helps to have a culinary flair to make them more appreciable, but this ignores the elephant in the room. The bigger problem is the fact that quinoa and buckwheat have served as staple crops for peoples in South America and Eastern Europe, respectively, for generations. Staple crops are, by nature, always energy-rich, they're high carbohydrate foods and therefore are not compatible with going keto.

Before really getting into the "meat" of it (heh), a special note should be made amount vegan "meats," as while they tend to be full of complete protein, many of them contain added carbohydrates and potentially unsavory additives, so it's important to check the ingredient list and nutritional content. Make sure the fat and protein are as close to normal meat as you can find, and that all the ingredients are things that you could potentially get right in a spelling bee. Nuts are also lauded as a source of protein, and while they are, oftentimes eating a lot of them can result in going over carbohydrate count, and they are not usually "complete" sources of protein.

Tofu and tempeh are two sides of the same coin, both are made from soybeans, and both are known for being bland and hard to get used to. Tempeh wins in that category because it's famous for being "bland, grainy, and slightly bitter," but with enough cooking knowledge, they are capable of amazing things, as they drink up the taste of whatever you cook with them, and are an excellent addition to soups and stews.

Nutritional yeast is also a criminally underrepresented vegan protein source. It has only one gram of net carb from carbohydrate, four grams of fiber, and nine grams of complete protein and a lot of it is fortified already with B12. It's the deactivated cousin of the fungal friend of humanity's that helps us make bread and has a taste that is weirdly reminiscent of cheese, so it's great for the former cheesemonger turned vegan.

Lastly, if fungi-dressed-up-as-cheese nor soy products are your thing, there's a third option for covering protein, but it's not "food" per se. Pea protein powder is a widely available supplement, and a complete protein to boot. So if you're having a hard time keeping the yeast and soy down, a pea protein shake mixed with MCTs might be just the thing.

Fat

For fat, you can be thankful that many vegan sources are unambiguously healthy -as long as they're minimally processed, and there are plenty of them, making getting your daily fat requirement simple. Olives, avocados, coconuts, nuts, and seeds in their various forms, and the oils extracted from them.

For saturated fat, the best (and most ethical) vegan source are coconuts and its oil. The reason "most ethical" is a point of contention is twofold – one is the inherent fact that many vegans are very concerned with ethics, given the nature of their diet. The other point is that palm oil production is infamously destructive in the area where it's typically farmed; southeastern Asia.

When cooking with fat, it's important to know the smoke point of your oils, if oil smokes, it's going toxic and producing free radicals, not something you want to be putting into your body. Non-vegans have a little more free reign with this, as they have access to fats like ghee, lard, and tallow, but given the veganism's restrictive nature, knowing how to cook with limited options is extremely important. Avocado oil is the shining star, having the highest heat amongst all cooking oils at 520 degrees Fahrenheit. So if you're deep frying some tofu fritters (is that a thing?) this would be the optimal choice. If you're looking to do lower-heat cooking, say sautéing garlic and onions before adding it to a sauce, virgin, unrefined olive or coconut oil is your better choice. These oils have a more delicate flavor and lower smoke point, so keeping them below that keeps its unique taste as well as keeping free radicals from causing a ruckus in your system.

A vegan keto diet might also be low in a number of other micronutrients, all of which can be found in the form of an appetizing supplemental capsule.

- ☒ Vitamin D: While it can be acquired from lightly toasting yourself by the pool, there are better ways of getting it. Namely, supplementation, but trace amounts can be found in mushrooms.

- ☒ Vitamin B12: This is another big hole in the vegan diet; because it can only come from animal sources and certain microorganisms. Many vegan foods are fortified with it, but it's also available in capsule form as well. Vitamin B12 necessary for proper digestion of fats and proteins, development of the myelin sheath that coats your neurons, and erythrogenesis; the production of red blood cells. It's important to say that there are some vitamin and mineral deficiencies that you can suffer through. Obviously they should be treated, but they don't hit you as hard as B12 deficiency, because B12 deficiency WILL kill you much faster.

- Vitamin C: You figure a vegan would have plenty of options to vitamin C, right? It's mainly found in plant sources, so there should be no trouble. Well, vitamin C is a delicate flower that is easily annihilated by heat and found a lot in fruit. And guess what you'll be eating as a vegan on keto? Not a lot of fruit and probably a lot of cooked vegetables. It's pretty easy to get this in the form of raw vegetables, most notably bell peppers and certain cruciferous vegetables; broccoli, cabbage, kale, and brussels sprouts.

- Calcium: Here's a big one; calcium is vital for bone strength and keeping the heart working. it's found easily in a number of animal products; dairy, cold water fatty fish, even eggshells if you're that much of an eccentric. If you're low on it, it's found in a variety of nuts and seeds, like sesame and tahini (tahini is a paste made from sesame seeds and oil) and flaxseed, and of course, in pill form.

- Zinc: This one is big for the boys, as it's essential for testosterone, but also for fighting off infection. It's somewhat more difficult to drain it from plant-based sources, so you may have to eat more to get the same amount. Again, it's found in nuts and seeds like sesame and tahini, pumpkin and sunflower seeds, and cashews. There's a trend here.

- ☒ Iron: Unless you like slipping into anemia, you need this. Again, it's harder to absorb non-heme (plant) iron than heme (animal) iron, so eat more than usual. Men are recommended to have 8, women 18 mg a day, but when you go vegan, it's closer to 12 and 33 a day. Common sources are spinach, olives, and tahini, sesame, chia, and pumpkin seeds.

- ☒ Omega-3s: One of the magic pills of the modern diet, and for most people comes from the oils of fish. Flaxseed oil and flaxseed oil tablets might be the thing to rush to, but they contain less EPA and DHA, which contain most of the more lauded health benefits of the omega-3 family. APA is in much higher quantities, but at the same time is not really the one that yields any health benefits. Instead, your body converts it to EPA and DHA. And very inefficiently, I might add. So, to get your fill of these two important fatty acids, consider seaweed/algae. It is indirectly the source of the omega-3s in fish, so go straight to the source and get it where the sardines get it.

So you want to go vegan, but aren't willing to start eating entirely akin to your herbivorous friends in the woods; nuts, seeds, and greens, and don't want to be making a paste of coconut oil and nutritional yeast like those of us in civilization, you'd like to keep your diet as close to "normal" as possible. Fear not, for the answer lies here. Many common foods that are not vegan have vegan replacement options to make transitioning just a little easier.

Milk

Milk is where both keto and vegans can proudly raise their banner, because it's not great for ketosis, given the carbohydrate count, and completely incompatible with veganism. There are a number of options to consider, and if buying them premade, remember to get the kind with no added sugars.

Coconut milk derives almost 100% of its calories from fat, a small amount of carbs and protein. It's a great source of medium chain triglycerides, which, if you remember, are often bottled and sold as a supplement as they are more easily used as energy than other forms of triglycerides.

Almond milk is the second runner up, with a higher ratio of carbs to fat, somewhere around 1:3, so for every gram of carb you get three of fat. It's relatively easy to make at home and packed with micronutrients, and it doesn't go under as much processing as soy milk, with the added benefit of there being no chance for it to screw with your hormones, and this applies to both men and women, as soy contains phytoestrogens.

Pea milk is another potential player, it contains an identical amount of protein as dairy milk, and tastes nothing like the mushy green orbs of deliciousness you may hate/love. The reason is that it's made from a flour that is then mixed with water and oil, keeping your protein and fat needs satisfied without throwing you into a bind with excess carbs.

Butter

When it comes to keto and vegan butter, there is really only one-stand in, and that's virgin coconut oil. It's spreadable and saturated just the same way, and is near identical in terms of fat content.

Yogurt

Yogurt is what happens when you introduce a certain bacteria in a certain liquid at a certain temperature and let it sit overnight, which is why there are perfectly viable options made from coconut, cashew, and almond that a ketogenic vegan can enjoy, so as long as there are no added sugars.

Cheese and cream cheese

There are a number of non-dairy cheeses made from tree nuts and soy. The best mimic for the taste of cheese, if not the texture, I retain to be nutritional yeast. Cream cheese substitutes can be made at home using cashews, but watch out for sugar content.

Eggs

Ground flaxseed – The most common substitute for eggs, when it comes to baking at least, is ground flaxseed mixed with water. If you've ever eaten whole flax seed, there's an almost waxy, gooey bit that forms as you pulverize it with your teeth. When you mix one tablespoon of flax with three of water, it serves the same binding purpose an egg does, imparting no flavor, merely serving in the same "structural" role. Chia seeds will also work for this, used in the same way with the same ratio.

Baking soda and vinegar – Two delicious stand-ins for eggs when you need to make something fluffier, which flaxseed is woefully under-equipped to do. The reaction they form makes whatever you're cooking bubbly and more airy. One teaspoon of baking soda to a tablespoon of vinegar is the usual ratio.

Silken Tofu does the opposite of baking soda and vinegar and is great for making foods denser than a neutron star. Like all tofu, it tastes like a glass of water would taste if you removed the flavor, so it's inoffensive and smoother than other tofu varieties. ¼ of a cup of it is about an egg.

The last thing to say is that there are a variety of premade egg substitutes on the market, and if you're considering them, remember to check the ingredients and nutritional value. The fat and protein ratio of both these premade substitutes and the ones you make in your kitchen will obviously not match that of a real egg, so keep your macronutrients in mind when using them.

Going back to our roots

While going keto and being vegan may seem difficult at first, with the right knowledge and a mind willing to experiment in the kitchen, it's easily attainable. Keep your diet rich in protein sources like tofu, nutritional yeast, and pea protein, eat plenty of healthy fats and remember to patch any holes in your dietary armor with any number of supplements. And keep your head up when trying to create the perfect egg or yogurt substitute, this part requires a bit of experimentation, and it's easy to get discouraged. "Fall down seven times, get up eight."

Chapter 10: Keto Myths

Keto myths are, unfortunately, nothing as colorful and hilarious as something like the mystical 13th labor of Hercules, where, using a keto diet, he shredded the excess fat from all the wine and bread to beat Thor for the first time in the Mr. Divinity contest; nor are they as backwoodsy as the legendary Florida Keto Ape, who breaks into your home, rifles through your pantry and steals all your MCTs and expensive olive oil. No, unfortunately, keto myths are more along the lines of "can too much protein at once kick me out of ketosis?" and "Can I go into ketoacidosis and die a horrible death?" Much, much drier, and require a lot more breakdown than the legend that the soma drank by Indo-Iranics was actually MCT oil. There is any number of different myths surrounding keto, but in this chapter, we'll try to cover some of the more conventional ones, the problems, and questions that are more likely to sew doubt in your mind.

1. Too much protein at once can kick me out of ketosis

We've started with one of the hardest ones, and it's tempting to believe, as your body uses the constituents of proteins, amino acids, along with a slew of other organic compounds to form glucose in the body. It's not as cut and dry as a yes or no, because the answer is closer to "no, but maybe yes. Depends on you man." To be frank, in both diabetics and nondiabetics, protein does not turn to sugar in any noticeable quantity, BUT it will spike insulin and glucagon. How much spikes your insulin depends on a number of factors – which is why the answer is GENERALLY "No if you're a healthy, non-diabetic adult," but everyone is different, so it's important that you learn how much protein you need. We'll cover the methodology of testing before we go into the why. This entire book, I've been praising 20% as the usual percentage, but that can be more or less, depending on you. This is one of the reasons why measuring your ketones is so bloody important.

Speaking of blood, a blood test strip is the best way to find your optimal protein requirement. Go on the keto diet for a week, keep your carbs at 5% and your protein at 20% and your fat at 75% of your daily intake. This should be enough to put you in ketosis. Then, test yourself. If you fall below 1.5 mmol/L, decrease your protein count by 5% and increase fat by 5% and test yourself again a week later. Repeat as needed and adjust your protein consumption accordingly.

Your protein need depends on a lot of things, to keep it short and sweet, men, especially active men need more. Your body composition matters, more muscular people will need more, and if you're trying to put on muscle, you'll need more. If you've been on keto a long time as well, your body is more used to using ketones, so the protein you consume is less likely to spike insulin to any degree. Lastly, there are factors outside your control that will determine protein consumption; namely genetics and insulin sensitivity. The more insulin sensitive you are, the less it interferes, and vice-versa.

2. You can go keto one day and go off it the next

Yo-yo dieting is one of the many characters in a metabolic rogue's gallery that our bodies just cannot tolerate. It leads to increased weight gain, increased risk of diabetes, and increased mortality. The jump from fat to skinny causes more stress on you than just carrying the extra weight. In the ketogenic diet, this is manifested in the person who eats keto one day and then carbohydrates the next and then back to keto the next day, forever and ever, ad infinitum. This is NOT how the keto diet works. The keto diet does best when the body adapts to it over time. The more adapted you are, the more efficient it gets at keeping off your weight, it burns more ketones, your brain gets more fed, everything gets more efficient. When you jump on and off it, you're basically putting your body through indecisive metabolic trauma and not getting the benefits of eating one way or the other. You might be going through symptoms of keto flu every time you try it for a day.

Everything in moderation is a life maxim that applies almost everywhere, almost. Obviously, you won't be eating a modest amount of carbohydrates, but that's not the point. Saturated fat, the solid-at-room-temperature fat that characterizes the fat in animal products, is good for you, good for hormones, HDLs, IN APPROPRIATE AMOUNTS. It's easy to go overboard with saturated fat because it's so delicious, and so many sources of fat are animal products. But the keto diet celebrates all fat, and monounsaturated fats are the unambiguous stars of health in the fat world. Enjoy a steak, enjoy salmon, butter, or lard, but keep it in moderation with plenty of healthy fats as well, because too much-saturated fat can lead to arterial clogging. If it's economically permissible, getting meat from locally sourced, humanely-treated animals and wild fish and game will always carry additional benefits.

No one can blame you if you read this book and think that I'm espousing that line of thinking, as I have continuously come back to the percentage of 75%-20%-5% of fat, protein, and carbs, over and over again. The first myth talked about particular protein requirements, as you can see, everyone is different. This also applies to carbohydrates, fats, and micronutrients. Some of us just don't need as much as others, or some of us need more. Say you're three or four weeks into the keto diet, you've tested yourself, and you're in deep ketosis, and, to top it all off, let's even say you're being a good little ketogenic and consuming MCTs. If you still feel like a hardboiled egg thrown across a greasy windshield (And do let me know how that feels) and your ketone levels are in the optimal range, and you're eating, say, 20 grams of carbs a day, it's perfectly possible that you're not getting enough of them. Up your carbohydrate intake by 10 grams or so and see how you feel, but remember to keep testing yourself and not go over the new limit you've set.

5. Ketosis is a risk factor for ketoacidosis

While it's true that your body has to enter ketosis before it goes into ketoacidosis, that doesn't mean that ketoacidosis is the logical conclusion to ketosis. Ketoacidosis is when your blood ketones rise so high you're in potentially life-threatening levels, which is a risk factor for those with diabetes mellitus, not ketogenic dieters, it's simply not a risk factor.

6. Ketosis is the ultimate, final way to lose weight

Though there are thousands of books claiming this, this isn't even close to true. Keto is a diet, and every diet doesn't work for everybody. Genetic conditions exist that make it hard for people's bodies to access and use the stored fat they have as fuel; others may simply not feel like following such a strict program. There are also risk factors if you do it wrong, muscle wasting, an increased psychological deviation that can lead to binge eating of unhealthy foods, which is why it's not the best long term solution for all of us, even most of us. It requires a certain discipline to make it work, for most of us it's a short-term solution that may work wonderfully when we're injured or don't have access to the gym for whatever reason. There's only one real "final" diet concept to swallow in case you need to drop weight, and that's calorie counting. If you can make sure that the calories you take in are less than those that you spend, you will lose weight. The problem with that is that it won't necessarily be the way you want, and it may be even more difficult for some of us than ketogenic dieting. Really, it's that, or to stop eating entirely.

7. Ketosis is a high protein diet

Let's get one thing cleared up; ketosis is a diet higher in protein than most people are probably used to because a lot more of our calories will be coming from animal products, which are high in protein. Having eggs and ham for breakfast and a steak for dinner may be the right kind of food for ketosis, but too much without tempering it with fat will simply cause the diet to fail and your ketosis to never occur. In addition, the chance of slipping into ketoacidosis for non-diabetics is very low; the chance increases if you eat too much protein when you're in deep ketosis. Amino acid breakdown into your blood could-potentially-maybe-might-possibly increase them even more, putting your blood at dangerously acidic levels.

8. Ketosis destroys your heart and valves

This is an easy one to see, because of the stark increase in fat and animal protein that people usually consume, but it's simply unfounded. When used correctly and weight is lost, as to what happens to those who follow the diet correctly, it lowers risk of heart disease. Furthermore, as long as you aren't consuming pork lard coated with butter, your triglyceride and LDL count should stay the same. Numerous studies have shown that low carb dieters versus low-fat dieters have had lower blood cholesterol and that the diet can effectively raise the HDL, "good" cholesterol, and improve signs like blood pressure.

9. Keto can cause flu-like symptoms

By now, you should be familiar with this one. This one is technically true, but only in the short-term adaptation period. Once there are a sufficient number of ketones in the bloodstream, and your brain has accepted them as its new fuel source, the fog should be lifted, and you'll be back to your old self.

10. Ketosis exacerbates fatty liver

If you can recall earlier in the book, one of the benefits of ketosis is that it has the power to loosen in particular the tough-to-get-at, really deep in, abdominal fat. Well, guess where the liver is? If you guessed the abdomen, I have good news! With this line of reasoning, we can pretty safely assume that the diet will do a fantastic job at helping alleviate fatty liver rather than making it worse. In fact, diets high in carbohydrates and alcohol are really the culprit in making it worse.

11. Ketosis carries out a systematic extermination of your gut flora

The source of this claim usually has something to do with the fact that certain keto-gone-wrong diets can be low in fiber, which wreaks havoc on everything stomach and below. In a well-balanced ketogenic diet, you should be getting tons of fiber, as though fiber is a carb, it's not digestible and therefore has no effect on blood sugar. If you're doing it right, you'll be eating plenty of fibrous vegetables. Some studies have shown that a ketogenic diet done right can be beneficial for gut flora, as carbohydrates can nourish some of the negative strains.

12. Any fat is good fat

The majority of the fat you should consume on the keto diet should be monounsaturated fat and a smaller amount of saturated fat, optimally from healthy, happy animals and wild fish. Putting a lot of polyunsaturated, highly processed corn, soybean, and vegetable oils is a waste of calories but not necessarily awful. There's no additional nutrients, and aren't high in MCTs, but good for hitting your macros if nothing else shows itself. It's also not an excuse to eat fast food hamburgers with no bun, because if the suspicious meat that doesn't decay after a year wasn't enough to keep you away, being cooked in artery-destroying trans-fat will.

And so it is written

The mythology surrounding the ketogenic diet is not like the exciting stories of the Theogony or Aeneid, and nowhere near as personally inspiring

(For most people, I'd estimate) but they are far more harmful and far more applicable in daily life. They spread misinformation about the diet, which can have a serious effect on those people who it might help who are looking to try it. For every person scared away by false knowledge, that's a person the keto diet could have helped.

Chapter 11: Good Foods

While theoretically you could approach keto and eat nothing but protein and greens powder mixed with water and washed down with olive and coconut oil, that is by far the worst and possibly silliest way to go about it. This chapter is dedicated to the best whole foods you can eat on keto, and those to avoid. It's not attempting to be a comprehensive or exhaustive list, but more as a guide to light your way and set you upon the path.

Fats and oils

- Extra-virgin olive oil – A strong tasting monounsaturated fat. Has serious benefits for reducing LDLs, blood pressure improves skin quality and could help with depression, Alzheimer's.
- Virgin coconut oil – In its refined form, saturated but still very healthy. It's full of MCTs, which are quickly tossed into the metabolic furnace as fuel, and has been connected with lower rates of inflammation.
- Avocado oil – Possibly the best oil for frying, as it has a 520-degree Fahrenheit smoke point. Monounsaturated, with a similar oleic acid content as extra virgin olive oil, giving it pro-cardiac, LDL lowering potencies.

- Lard - Not deserving of its reputation as an artery-clogging cardiac nightmare, from the right pigs and rendered from scraps at home, lard can be high in monounsaturated fat and full of omega-3s

- Grass-fed butter and ghee - Keyword here is grass-fed. Grass-fed steps all over grain-fed health wise - more vitamins, conjugated linoleic acid, and omega-3s. In case you aren't a nutritionist, know that conjugated linoleic acid has a smorgasbord of random health benefits, supporting bone health, muscle development, and soothing inflammation. And what is ghee, you may ask? Well, I'm glad you asked. Ghee is clarified butter - butter with the milk solids strained out, with a similar nutrient profile and fantastic for high-heat cooking.

Meat, poultry, and seafood

- Fatty fish - You want to go heavy on the fish that looks like it can't fit into its pants anymore, but keep it wild. Wild, fatty fish - think salmon, trout, sardines, kippers, herring, and tuna, is the most famous and abundant source of omega-3s we know of, along with high-quality fat and protein. Omega-3s curb inflammation, contribute to brain and heart health and keep the eyeballs working. They also contain large amounts of vitamin D, and, if canned fish is your thing, calcium from the bones. If you're concerned about mercury content, go small with tiny canned fish. Because they are the wimps of the ocean and are low on the food chain, they don't contain huge chunks of mercury (as a way of speaking) like the bigger fish, such as tuna.

- Grass-fed beef/local beef - Depends if you want to get up early enough in the morning to go to your local farmer's market. Grass-fed beef contains higher amounts of omega-3s, vitamin B and E, beta-carotene, and conjugated linoleic acid than corn-fed beef. It also contains less fat - to make up for that, choose the fattier cuts like rib or chuck cuts. Local beef depends on your farmer, but usually small-time farmers have healthier, happier animals who pass this benefit up to you. Talk to your local farmer and see what he feeds his cows to get a better idea of what you're getting.

- Pasture-raised pork: There's a trend amongst meat; and that's when the animal is happier and healthier, it comes out tasting better and better for you — what a strange idea. Not only does their meat have a better flavor with a higher fat content than factory raised pork, but their fat is also rich in vitamin D, and omega-3s and their meat isn't contaminated with antibiotics and growth hormone.

⊠ Pasture-raised chicken: Consider buying dark meat, as it's more nutritious, higher in fat, and cheaper. Like the other humanely-raised meat, pasture-raised chicken is higher in omega-3s and lower in omega-6s, with higher counts of selenium and B3 than its conventional, factory farmed cousin. B3 is important for energy and digestion, and selenium is a potent antioxidant.

⊠ Pasture-raised eggs: The spawn of pasture-raised chickens, and most definitely a meat despite people trying to categorize them as "dairy." Eggs have been called "nature's perfect food," and it's not hard to see why. They come prepackaged with a durable outer container, a great percentage of fat and protein can be used in nearly everything, and it's easy to eat five or six of them without feeling like death. Not being raised in what can be described as a hellish dungeon for chickens, pasture-raised eggs have oodles more omega-3 and vitamin E than their prison-spawned equivalents.

- Bone broth: Not technically a meat, but what happens when you suspend gelatin, protein, and fat in water. The collagen has great benefits for your skin, nails, and joints, and make sure to add plenty of salt for both electrolytes and to make it taste less like a barnyard.

A note on meat and seafood: Almost any pasture-raised, humanely slaughtered meat is going to be good on the ketogenic diet, but it's not a necessity. It can get expensive quickly, especially if you're an athlete. In that case, consider supplements for the micronutrients and omega-3s you'll be missing. In addition, other meats, such as mutton and lamb, chevron (goat meat), offal, and veal are all fantastic choices when eaten in the right proportions. You may have noticed that shellfish was omitted - it appears shellfish is slightly higher in carbohydrates, depending on the type eaten, than other kinds of seafood, which is why it can't be recommended in earnest as a great food. It can, of course, be a part of a healthy ketogenic diet, as long as you make sure that you limit how much of it you eat.

Nuts, Seeds, Legumes, etc.:

There's not really an easy category for these guys, so they go alone. They contain everything in your mixed nuts jar - peanuts, almonds, sesame, sunflower seeds, so on and so forth. All of them can be made into jars of butter at home with a blender and some grit. All of them are rich sources of monounsaturated fat, fiber, and protein, so, in a quest to not repeat myself too often, only the micronutrient profiles and other benefits will be highlighted. Also, not all of them will be listed, because that would take probably way more space than necessary, only the more common specimens.

- Peanuts: Minerals like copper and manganese
- Almonds: Biotin and vitamin E
- Sunflower seeds: A combination of the two lads above them, rich in Vitamin E and copper.
- Walnuts: When consumed skin on, flavonoids and other antioxidants. Omega-3s and copper are found in the flesh of the walnut.
- Sesame: Omega-3s, copper, and manganese, which is why it was often referred to as the "eastern peanut." The last part is made up.

There are obviously hundreds of breeds of nuts in existence, and it would be akin to Sisyphus and his boulder to list them all, but in general, nuts are a fantastic source of nutrition for the keto dieter and a worthy addition to their nutritional arsenal for both snacking and cooking.

Most fruit is right out because of its high sugar content, but there are two "stars."

- ☒ Avocado: If you didn't see this coming, you might need to make sure you can actually read. Avocado has so many health benefits the rest of this chapter could be dedicated to it, but I'll resist and give a basic overview. Avocados are full of fiber and monounsaturated fat, vitamins K, C, B, and E, and tons of potassium. They're also filling, VERY self-contained, and versatile. Delicious in protein shakes!

- ☒ Olives: Olives have a very similar nutritional content to olive oil. Who'd have thought it? Monounsaturated fat, antioxidants, and vitamin E come pre-packed in a nice little orb. If you're watching the sodium intake putting a hard limit on them isn't such an unwise idea.

In this context, vegetables in fruit are sort of opposite. Low carb vegetables are absolute darlings, and eat as many as you can in as many varieties as you can. Because most vegetables are inherently low carb and good for you, we're going to have a similar policy and pick only a handful of true standouts. If there's something not on the list here and your body desires of it, look up the nutritional information to assure it fits your carb goals, and enjoy. It will be said here and nowhere else that every single vegetable is full of fiber, so I don't sound like a broken record.

- Tomatoes: Not only are they good for throwing at bad stage actors, but fresh tomatoes are also delicious raw, cooked, or in a sauce or soup. Look to our red friends for micronutrients like vitamins C and K, (vitamin C when raw) potassium, and B9, the experimental sci-fi name for folate.

- Brassica family vegetables: Hold your horses, before you start throwing whole cabbages at me, think of this as an experiment in efficiency. ALL brassica (cabbage) family veggies are good for you. This includes cabbage (wow!) cabbagini (a custom word that means "small cabbage" - brussels sprout) broccoli, kale, and cauliflower. All of these veggies are chock full of antioxidants, vitamin C, vitamin K, potassium, and iron. A word of warning - there's a chance in poisoning yourself if you eat too much kale from the huge bomb of vitamin K. As a way to enjoy these foods that typically might make adults and children cringe, try serving them up with a huge scoop of butter or bacon. Really eases the bitterness.

- Spinach: Obligatory Popeye, the Sailor Man joke, followed up with actual nutritional information. Famed for its iron and ability to spontaneously generate massive amounts of muscular power in nautical tough guys, it also has plenty of folic acids, calcium, and phytonutrients. If you're anything like me, you'll be tempted to knock on your dentist's door and ask him why your teeth are failing because of the weird grittiness on your teeth. That's a certain type of acid found in broken down spinach – not harmful, but if it's in a bad mood it might stop you from absorbing some of that iron, so give it a spritz of lemon or lime juice before you uppercut Brutus into the stratosphere.

- Eggplant: Eggplant is interesting, it's not necessarily packed with any nutrients besides the obligatory fiber and medium dose of manganese, and it should be salted an hour before consumed because of a compound related to nicotine makes it taste bitter, but it's a potentially powerful tool for keeping you full. The reason being is that it drinks up the flavors of whatever you cook it in, so it could be filled with nutritious and filling olive oil and tomato sauce or whatever else you choose to be its vessel.

- ☒ Asparagus: If there's any vegetable best suited for pretending you're in an ancient Greek phalanx wielding a *dory* (spear) at the dinner table, it's asparagus. Besides for LARPing, asparagus is useful for being filled with vitamins A, C, E, and K. And as easily as the Hellenic *dory* fends off Persian armies and reduces near-eastern influence, asparagus' high antioxidant content fends off free radicals and reduces oxidative stress.

Dairy

The big kid on campus of dairy, milk, is technically acceptable, but probably not the best choice as it does have quite a bit of sugar per serving. The good news is that in two of its mutant forms, cheese, and yogurt, it's much lower in lactose but still full of protein, calcium, and vitamin D. If you haven't figured it out by now, go with the full-fat varieties, for reasons of satiety.

- ☒ Cheese: The enzymy, degenerate, delicious form of milk. It's filling and full of protein and healthy fat and almost no carbs. It's almost like a form of curdled meat product in terms of nutritional value – and contains calcium. Whole fat mozzarella cheese sticks are an excellent snack, roughly the equivalent of a boiled egg if you don't feel like boiling it and destroying half of it as you peel it.

- ☒ Yogurt: Here's a classic joke originating from the central Asian steppe, where yogurt originated: What do you get when you leave your milk in a leather pouch for too long? Yogurt! Obviously, these steppe nomads had a poorly developed sense of humor. Yogurt has a few more carbs but has the upside of being a probiotic food. As mentioned in the "joke" earlier, yogurt was found to have originated from old milk left in a leather pouch carried by steppe peoples, and was probably a cozy home for Lactobacillus, as it quickly migrated to the milk to form yogurt. The lactobacillus colonizes your gut, and can positively affect everything from muscular pain to mental health. As a rule, pick strained – or Greek – yogurt, as its higher in protein and lower and carbs. Much like mozzarella sticks, strained yogurt is usually sold prepackaged in containers with all of its nutritional information on the side.

- Heavy cream: Finally, our dreams of coffee half-cream half-coffee are realized. Heavy cream is great for meeting our fat goals and is a tasty addition to scores of dishes.

- Sour cream/Creme fraiche: For the Tex-Mex lovers, I have kept you from your beans, rice, and tortillas. But I have bestowed upon you the privilege of your delicious sour cream condiment, as it is essentially all fat. The same goes for creme fraiche, actually slightly higher in fat content than sour cream, and goes great with eggs.

Snacks:

- Pork rinds: Keto chips can take two forms, and one of them is a bit of deep-fried pork skin. Pork rinds are a great source of protein and fat, far more filling than regular potato chips, and can be made at home.

- Parmesan chips: The other form of the keto chip and possibly one of the tastiest culinary innovations in recent years. They have the same nutrition as parmesan/romano cheese, high in protein and fat, and are simple to make at home. Probably less of a time investment than the pork rinds, really.

- Dehydrated vegetables: If you own a dehydrator, rejoice. You can dry any number of leafy greens and other vegetables in huge amounts and end up with much smaller amounts of snacks the next day. When made at home, you can customize their flavor however you want and are far cheaper than the ones made in the store. In addition, you can trust that there are no suspicious unpronounceable additives. Dehydrated vegetables retain all the nutrition of regular vegetables, as the low heat of dehydration isn't enough to denature them. They can also be done with an oven on the lowest setting and enough patience.

Drinks:

- ☒ Water: You will die in three days max without water. You are 70% water. That should be enough to get you to drink it. It's absolutely necessary for all life functions, it's refreshing, and keeps hunger at bay. If you need a little bit of extra flavor, try adding lemon, lime, grapefruit, or cucumber to your water and refrigerating it overnight.

- ☒ Tea and coffee: As long as they're unsweetened, you can have your caffeine. One of the keto rages is bulletproof coffee – I see no reason why the same idea can't theoretically work with tea as well. Try blending in a bit of butter into your tea if you're used to taking it with milk for an energy boost, and report back to me on how it tasted.

Foods to avoid on this diet tends to be a little more apparent if you actually read this book. A general rule of good nutrition is to avoid processed foods, sugar, and trans fat. Keto takes all these rules and turns its furious gaze on starchy carbohydrates and fruit as well.

Fats:

- Polyunsaturated fat: These are fats like your typical cooking oils - corn oil, peanut oil, canola oil, and soybean oil. There's nothing particularly bad about these oils - they are heavily processed and contain less nutrients than monounsaturated fats like avocado, olive, or coconut oils. Their strongest upside is they're cheap. They technically are fine if you need your fat for the day, but there are much better choices, with more omega-3s and linoleic acid.
- Trans Fat: Now this guy is definitely a shady character. Trans fats are found in processed foods; fast food burgers, pizza, and all its other deviant forms. Trans fats have been

solidly linked to an increased risk of heart disease, so keep these out of your diet at any cost.

- ☒ Processed meat: Hold your horses, I know your farmer friend "processes" chickens and makes salami, but that's not we're referring to. We're talking about things like chicken nuggets, frozen pre-prepared meats, anything you get from a fast food establishment, and mass-produced hotdogs, jerky, and cold cuts. There's been a solid link between processed food and colon cancer from the preservation agents. There's also the reality that most of it is full of trans fat and unsavory additives. In small amounts, more traditionally prepared cured meats, like pancetta, nitrate-free bacon, serrano ham, and the like aren't dangerous, but they should be part of a larger diet and not the main source of protein.

- ☒ Breaded meat: Yes, I'm aware that the mob will come at me with pitchforks and torches for this one, but it's true. Breaded meat is delicious - cutlets, fried chicken, schnitzel, and while it is usually deep fat fried, the breading on it is plain unnecessary and bad for a ketogenic diet.

Starches

There's virtually no point in breaking down why you shouldn't have starch on this diet, it should be obvious to you, and if it's not one or both of us needs to reassess our life choices because either you can't read or I can't write or both. Pasta, bread, rice, beans, quinoa, sweet and regular potatoes are all carbohydrate-rich and forbidden. There are times when eating them is acceptable - athletes following the ketogenic diet could get the athletic rush they need from them, but if you're not doing that particular breed of keto, avoid them.

Fruits

See above and replace "starch" with "fruit." Fruit is high in sugar, and that's how trees tricked us into eating it long, long ago. Fruit can, of course, be part of a healthy diet, but it's better to avoid to stay in keto. There are exceptions - olives and avocados of course, and tomato if you're that breed of pedantic who insists on categorizing it with vegetables. Berries, eaten in controlled amounts, can be okay, but okay is not necessarily enough to recommend them, and it's very easy to go overboard. Because of this, they err closer to the side of "don't eat" than "eat."

Vegetables

Avoid anything starchy. This includes potatoes of all breeds, yuca/cassava, breadfruit, corn, squashes. When in doubt, consult nutritional information. Other than that, all non-starchy vegetables have two thumbs up for keto.

Sugars, sweeteners, desserts, etc.

Another no-brainer. Avoid sugar, honey, maple syrup, and artificial sweeteners. Artificial sweeteners have conflicting data - some have displayed insulin spikes, others don't. In my mind, it's better to avoid all of them to avoid the risk altogether. And as tempting as it may to shove a cannoli down your throat the first week, these sugary desserts are also to be avoided like the plague.

Snacks

Things like cheese puffs, potato chips, and candy should all be avoided. Most snacks are made from cheap carbohydrates, and the ones that are meat-based are often more or less suspicious. Stay vigilant when selecting things like store-bought vegetable chips as well.

Drinks:

Soda, sweet tea or coffee, sports drinks, milkshakes are immediately on the chopping block. They're all, by necessity, full of carbohydrates. If you're a fan of kvass, a malted drink from eastern Europe, that is basically unfermented beer and made from bread, so that's to be avoided. Alcoholic beverages in most forms are included too, cocktails are elaborate dressings of liquor and sugar, wine is rotten grape juice, and beer is what happens when you leave your grain harvest bubbling in a metal tank for too long, so those are all out as well.

Conclusion

When this book was written, one of the goals was to be the single, most condensed, easy and fun to read book on the keto diet, covering everything from the very basics, to the science, to how to manage your lifestyle and activity with it, and what to eat while on it. You can go to hundreds of different papers and hundreds of articles to find the precise lifestyle information and scientific knowledge that you need, but hopefully, after compartmentalizing this, you won't have to.

The other goal of this book was to instill a sense of independence into the reader - to give a thorough and sufficient explanation in simple language. Additionally, its aim was to answer any further questions you might have based off the reasoning and explanations you gained from devouring (not literally, good source of fiber though) this book. An old expression says "give a man a fish, he's fed for a day. Teach a man to fish, and he's fed for a lifetime."

It's obvious that keto isn't for everyone - there's more than one way to do it, and it's, by nature, very restrictive. It requires patience, testing, and the ability to suffer through a few weeks of the flu-but-not-the-flu, but if you stick through it, it will come with rewards. Maybe you were trying to wrestle better control over a chronic disease, maybe you were interested in a fast-track way of changing your body composition, of shedding excess weight without having to do hours of grueling cardio and keeping your maxes in the gym, or maybe you were simply trying it out to see what the fuss is about. Whatever reasons you had when picking up this book, I hope that you found what you were looking for.

Finally, if you found this book useful in any way, a review on Amazon is always appreciated!